BOOK DESCRIPTION

Bad habits are not easy to break, but it's not impossible. To break a bad habit, we have to replace it with another habit, a good one. When it comes to bad eating habits, it's quite feasible to develop healthy habits that will help you reach good end results that will make you feel proud of yourself.

To deal with bad habits, we have to first identify and acknowledge them. This book aims to help people who are unable to lose or manage their weight due to the bad habits that they acquire. In Part 1 and Part 2, this book will help you understand the real reasons behind weight gain, the importance of maintaining the right body weight, help you identify bad habits, and provide examples of good habits that you can easily adopt.

Part 3 includes a habits workbook in which you can keep a record of your progress as well as your challenges. The book also offers you a 30-day workout challenge in Part 4, as well as several 10-minute workouts that you can easily do at home. Finally, part 5 includes a long list of healthy, tasty, and easy to prepare recipes to motivate you to cook your own healthy meals.

The journey to weight loss isn't as hard as everyone thinks. You just need to make some adaptations to your lifestyle and switch to healthy alternatives. This will not only result in losing weight but improving your overall physical and mental health as well.

BAD HABITS

Weight Loss Mentality

Erik M. Rosales

© Copyright 2021 - All rights reserved.

The content contained within this book may not be reproduced, duplicated or transmitted without direct written permission from the author or the publisher.

Under no circumstances will any blame or legal responsibility be held against the publisher, or author, for any damages, reparation, or monetary loss due to the information contained within this book, either directly or indirectly.

Legal Notice:

This book is copyright protected. It is only for personal use. You cannot amend, distribute, sell, use, quote or paraphrase any part, or the content within this book, without the consent of the author or publisher.

Disclaimer Notice:

Please note the information contained within this document is for educational and entertainment purposes only. All effort has been executed to present accurate, up to date, reliable, complete information. No warranties of any kind are declared or implied. Readers acknowledge that the author is not engaged in the rendering of legal, financial, medical or professional advice. The content within this book has been derived from various sources. Please consult a licensed professional before attempting any techniques outlined in this book.

By reading this document, the reader agrees that under no circumstances is the author responsible for any losses, direct or indirect, that are incurred as a result of the use of the information contained within this document, including, but not limited to, errors, omissions, or inaccuracies.

TABLE OF CONTENTS

INTRODUCTION

It is important to understand the power of habits. You can easily use your habits for good or bad, but identifying your own personal habits and changing them towards the positive end of the scale will serve you well as a firm foundation on which to build your healthier lifestyle from scratch.

Developing healthy eating habits forms the cornerstone of a healthy life, and the impact this will have on our health and well-being is crucial. You cannot live a healthy life if you continue to indulge in habits that are detrimental to your health and well-being. If you constantly overeat when you feel emotional, you are going to sabotage any efforts towards losing weight. If you always procrastinate when you are under a little pressure, you are going to put off the things that are important and never achieve what you really want to achieve.

Habits can be both good and bad, but you can control them for yourself and use them for your greater good.

One of the things that most of us wish for ourselves is to be healthy. Health is the most important thing you can have in life. Many people believe that being healthy, slim, and fit is hard to achieve. Actually, focusing on health, in general, is far easier than most people think. However, for this to happen, for you to become healthier, you need to realize that changes need to be made. You need to make decisions to change your diet, lose weight, or start an exercise regime. However, motivation is often short-lived, and learning to extend it is key.

A healthy lifestyle requires you to develop long-term healthy eating habits, and this is something that most people struggle with, simply because they do not know where to start. This struggle often contributes to loss of motivation, and when motivation is gone, disappointment quickly takes over. Feeling this way tends to pull us back to our old habits and behaviors, along with a dose of self-loathing as a result of the perceived failure.

Of course, not achieving something is not necessarily a failure, but allowing your motivation to desert you, and not doing anything about getting it back, is something that needs to be addressed.

Understanding that your new habits cannot be developed overnight is vital. It takes time to create them, and it takes energy to practice them. Only after many regular repetitions can they become a part of your regular behavioral pattern. However, creating healthy habits does not need to be hard work, and it is often simply a matter of adding a new pattern of behavior to your existing, well-established behavior. This is a very simple way of managing your well-being, although no one can deny that it takes time and effort.

If you carry on doing what you have always done, you will get what you always had. It is that simple. Finding excuses for being too busy, and putting blame on others for the inability to have the life you want, will not bring you success. Developing new and healthy habits can only start, and be maintained, by having the determination to succeed and understanding how your new behavior can change your life. It is not about relying on other people or circumstances but about creating the circumstances that you want to live in. You have the power in your own hands, and you need to open your heart and your eyes to the fact that the only person who can sabotage your efforts is you, and the only person who can help you onwards is also you.

To achieve what you want, whatever it is, you have to start with creating new habits. The best way to achieve this is to add new behavior to your existing habits, and soon afterward you will notice that your new behavior is turning into a new habit, replacing the old behavioral pattern. How to follow this part of the process will be discussed later on in this book, but for now, simply be mindful of the fact that old habits can be changed and new ones can be added.

We all have habits, and they help us get through life. However, a habit is more than just something we do often. There is normally a trigger that starts the action and a pay-off that gives us pleasure. The problem comes when it is a short-term pleasure that is bad for us in the long run. For example, the trigger for eating something unhealthy may be anything from feeling depressed or bored to passing a vending machine. The pay-off is the short-term "high" that sugary or fatty food can give, but that is soon replaced by a "low" when you realize you are putting on weight and do not have the energy you need.

One of the major problems in developing healthy habits is that the pay-off is usually more immediate and obvious for unhealthy habits. For instance, an immediate sugar rush from unhealthy food as opposed to the long-term benefits of healthy eating. Or lounging on the sofa, watching your favorite TV program, rather than going out for a run in the middle of a winter's day, when the weather is cold and it is dark outside.

This is the reason why it is vital to be clear about the benefits of your healthy habits. When you know why something is going to benefit you, it is easier to stay focused upon achieving it as a goal. Understanding the benefits of making any sort of change in life can help you overcome the lure of unhealthy but instant gratification.

The effect of your habits on your everyday life is enormous and should never be underestimated. Most of your behaviors are determined by the long-term habits you have repeated a number of times before, and as such, they have become your way of life.

Some habits are good and others are bad, but all of them are equally important as they create the foundation on which your daily routines are built. The routines that you develop affect all areas of your life and play a significant role in your health, finances, relationships, etc. The key is to determine which habits are damaging to you and which ones benefit you. By doing that, you can change the damaging ones and increase your focus on the beneficial ones.

Most of the habits you currently have were developed a long time ago. They have been formed through consistency and repetition, to the point where you probably do not even realize you are doing them. That is the reason why, even when the habits are not doing you any favors, you make excuses for their existence in order to protect them. You feel loyal to them, and you find it hard to let them go. They are part and parcel of your life and who you are to a large degree.

I understand this. Let's be honest; you have spent months, years, and even decades in their company. You have been living with them, sleeping with them, and then they became your family and your best friends. It is hard to imagine living your life without them, and when you start to try and change them, it is normal to feel a little nervous or even slightly lost. The good news is that this will pass.

Of course, I agree that creating new and healthy habits, and getting rid of your old and unhealthy habits, is not always easy when life is so busy and terribly stressful. But, focusing on what really matters to you will help you develop a different type of mindset, and it is this mindset that will allow you to overcome challenges in your new healthier lifestyle plan.

Your new mindset will also support you in creating new patterns of behavior and provide you with an opportunity to make your body healthier, working towards a more fulfilling life. Feeling good about yourself will encourage you to embrace the change, and as a result, you will notice your confidence beginning to soar. When that happens, anything is possible.

It is important to remember that the aim of establishing

healthy habits is not to restrict yourself but to enhance your life beyond what it is right now. This is a life built on healthy habits, containing all the great ingredients required for health and happiness, including healthy thoughts, healthy attitude, healthy words, and healthy actions. Becoming healthier is not all about eating more fruit and vegetables and moving your body more; it is about loving who you are and making time for yourself too. It is an entire package deal that needs to be embraced fully if you want the effects to snowball into something that makes a real difference in your life.

I would like to remind you that the perfect start for creating a healthy eating habit that leads towards a new behavior is to visualize where you want to be and why. Visualize your endpoint. Let your vision be your guide. Imagine the end result, and work towards the beginning. By doing this, you will subconsciously create a path in your mind that will take you to your goal. It might seem like you are working backward in many ways, but you are already motivated by this point because you have seen what it will look like and feel like if you achieve your goal. That is the ultimate motivation.

If your goal is to have less stress and more relaxation, less anxiety and more calmness, less illness and more health, less worry and more joy, then your action plan must include creating a lifestyle that will prioritize things that can give you relaxation, calmness, health, and joy. This includes developing healthy lifestyle habits, healthy eating habits, a healthy relationship with yourself and others, and understanding your own needs.

Taking only one small step at a time is enough. Often, it is more than enough. Each step will move you forward and bring your goals closer to you.

Now, imagine if you decided to make just one small change in your behavior every day of the week. That would be 365 changed habits this time next year. Would your life be different in any way if you did this? What do you think?

Okay, maybe changing your behavior every day sounds too overwhelming. If this is the case, then focus on making one small change in your behavior once per week. That will be 52 changes in your behavior this time next year. Do you think that making 52 changes in your behavior, and creating 52 new habits, will improve your life? Of course, it will.

Can you think of the ways in which your life could improve by doing this? I am sure you can think of many, and those changes will turn into even bigger benefits the more energy you focus on them.

The most important aspect of your habits is to remember that they are not fixed. All your habits were created because they served a purpose at the time. Every single habit you have right now was consciously created, unconsciously accepted, and it became a part of your life because you carried on doing it. You can change the unwanted habits that work against you, and swap them with those that work for you.

In addition, you can change them any time you wish and anyway you like, but in order for you to benefit from them, you need to make sure that your new habits fit your life, accommodate your needs, and take you down the path that leads towards your goals.

Another thing to remember is that when it comes to creating a new habit, you need to make your new behavior your point of focus. Stop searching for excuses that could prevent you from doing your best.

I know that working on developing a new habit, which eventually becomes your standard behavior, often seems like a difficult task to do. And it is especially hard when you are at the initial stage of creating a change. But focusing on your new behavior has to be on the top of your priority list, and it has to stay there until it becomes a habit, despite the difficulties you might be experiencing on the way. Your efforts will pay off at the end when you notice that your new habits are responsible for bringing many positive changes in your life.

Ultimately, I would like you to remember that you are in control of your behavior. You are in control of all your actions. It is only you who can make the change, and any change that you make will eventually make a big difference in your life, in the way you feel, and of course, in your future.

PART 1: WEIGHT LOSS

We are in the early days of a new year and weight loss is obviously on the bucket list of a number of people for different reasons.

Many people are looking to drop the holiday weight they gained from spending time with loved ones munching on a lot of food that might have been unhealthy. Others are looking to drop the weight they've gained from neglecting their bodies due to the trying nature of the previous year. Whatever the reasons are, you are most likely reading this book because just like others, you are trying to lose some weight.

While there are many quick fixes and solutions, it has been proven that the healthiest way to lose weight is by incorporating little everyday habits that can make all the difference.

When many people think of weight loss, the first thing that comes to mind is physical exertion. Weight loss conjures thoughts of hours spent in the gym or running on tracks.

While this is great, it is not a true reflection of weight loss habits. If it were, it would mean that if you go through a period when you cannot physically exert yourself as you used to, you would not only stop losing weight, you will gain weight.

This is where passive weight loss habits come into play. They ensure that even on days when you do not have the time to work out, you can still lose weight or maintain weight loss.

Obesity levels amongst people are certainly higher than they have ever been in history. This trend has spread throughout the world. People are gaining weight at excessive rates. But the big question is, why? What is it that is really causing people to gain weight?

The quick answer is to blame it on junk food, and that would be the logical answer. There are so many food manufacturing companies that are creating junk foods that are not healthy for people to consume.

Junk foods are basically processed foods that have been altered from their natural state. Common junk foods contain added pesticides, preservatives, flavorings, sugars, salts, seasonings, and all kinds of things that are bad for our health.

Unnatural foods will cause you to feel unnatural. In other words, they will cause you to feel symptoms of stress, anxiety, irritation, irregular heartbeats, and more. Even though these symptoms may be natural in some life circumstances, when they are caused simply by food, then they are unnatural.

The Real Reason

We know junk food is the cause of most health problems in America and other developed countries. Until government agencies ban junk foods from being sold in the supermarkets, they are always going to be there and people will always buy them.

It is no surprise to ordinary citizens that junk food is bad for them when they see it in the supermarkets. They know cookies, cakes, pizza, and fried foods are just going to make them feel lousy after they eat them. But they continue to eat these foods anyway. So again, why?

The real reason has to do with stress more than anything else. People live such stressful lives in the modern age. They have to worry about making a living, taking care of their kids, and so on. It gets to a point where they really have no time to relax and feel comfortable at all.

People in stressful situations tend to form bad habits in order to relieve their stress. One of the biggest habits people develop is binge eating junk food in order to gain temporary relief.

However, the unnatural chemicals and additives in those foods will raise their stress levels even higher in the long run. So instead of treating the problem, junk food just makes it worse.

Control the Eating

It is important that you understand the difference between emotional eating and regular eating. For example, if you are on a typical diet and you are able to control what you eat, this is regular eating.

When someone eats to relieve their stress and anxiety, this is emotional eating. Even someone who regularly sticks to a healthy diet regime could find themselves eating poorly if they are stressed. This is the inner demon that you must learn to fight.

So, how does someone gain the discipline to control their eating under stressful situations? The first step is to try and distance yourself from all unhealthy foods.

This means no filling your kitchen cupboards with junk food from the supermarket. Only fill your house with healthy foods. After all, if there are no unhealthy foods in your house, then you won't be tempted to cheat.

Now if you are away from your house, like at work, then you might find vending machines nearby that will tempt you into eating poorly. These are always hard to resist for someone under distress.

Fortunately, there are certain types of foods you can eat beforehand that will help limit your cravings and relieve stress:

- Avocados – These are fruits that contain folic acid and vitamin B6. These nutrients have been scientifically proven to reduce stress levels by helping the central nervous system function well. They also contain potassium, which regulates blood pressure.
- Salmon – This type of fish is very high in omega-3 fatty acids, which can elevate you into a good mood. These acids also keep your heart strong, especially if your cortisol levels are high. These stress hormones get released under

pressure and cause damage to your heart if they remain high. Omega-3s will prevent this.

- Broccoli – This vegetable is a good source of Vitamin C, which strengthens the immune system. When you feel stress and anxiety, it can put a burden on your immune system. It will even make you susceptible to colds and flu bugs, so supporting immune system function can help you stay healthy.
- Almonds – These nuts are loaded with magnesium, which is a mineral that lowers cortisol levels. This will calm down the nervous system when it starts feeling stressed out. You will even sleep better as a result of eating these, which will then help you in other ways as well.

These are the four foods you should always have on hand with you, whether you are at work, school, or wherever.

Two of these foods are so simple to carry that you don't even need to cook them. As for the salmon and broccoli, just cook them beforehand and bring them with you in a Tupperware container.

Now, every time you start feeling stressed out during the day, go ahead and eat a little bit of these foods. You don't necessarily have to eat bites from all of them, although that wouldn't hurt. If you are under time constraints and don't have time to eat, then almonds would be the best food to munch on.

Almonds can conveniently be eaten from your desk at work or anywhere. Since they lower cortisol levels, this will ultimately be what you need to keep your stress under control. Then when you have your next lunch break, go ahead and eat the rest of the foods to further calm yourself down.

Now, you can still eat other fruits and vegetables if these mood friendly foods don't fill you up. But just remember to stay away from all processed foods because they will reverse the positive feelings you have already gained from the healthier mood foods.

Eventually, you will start to develop a habit of controlling your mood through healthy eating every time you feel stressed out. Then it will become a routine for you, which means you will have successfully turned a bad habit into a good one.

Importance of Losing Weight

If you are obese or overweight, you may have a higher risk of developing the following:

- Heart disease
- High blood pressure
- Stroke
- Type 2 diabetes
- Osteoarthritis
- Back pain (NHS Choices, 2019)

Increased Metabolic Health

Metabolic syndrome is characterized as having common risk factors for heart disease, type 2 diabetes, and obesity. These include high blood sugar levels, low levels of HDL "good" cholesterol, high levels of LDL "bad" cholesterol, abdominal obesity, and high blood pressure. Fortunately, many of these risk factors can be eliminated or improved through better lifestyle and nutritional changes. An important factor behind these issues is insulin. Insulin plays a vital role as far as metabolic disease and diabetes go.

Improved Kidney Function

Another common issue among the health community is kidney stones. The most common cause of gout and kidney stones is elevated phosphorus levels, oxalate, calcium, and uric acid in the body. This is often related to obesity, dehydration, bad genetics, sugar consumption, and alcohol consumption. Luckily, the lifestyle changes discussed here can help you combat these risk factors and improve your kidney function.

HEALTH RISKS OF BEING OVERWEIGHT AND OBESE

Type 2 Diabetes

This disease occurs when the blood sugar level becomes higher than normal. According to studies, about 80% of individuals afflicted with type 2 diabetes are overweight (Mandal, 2014). What makes diabetes such a serious disease is that it is a major cause of stroke, heart disease, kidney diseases, amputation, and even blindness.

Sleep Apnea

This is when an individual stops breathing for short periods while sleeping. Being overweight or obese is a risk factor. Why? This is because the fat stored in the neck area makes the air pathway smaller. In addition, the fat could also cause inflammation. Sleep apnea should not be taken lightly because it can also result in heart failure.

Metabolic Syndrome

If you have a large waistline, a low HDL cholesterol level, a higher than normal triglyceride level, high blood pressure, and higher fasting blood sugar, you are a likely candidate for this disease. As mentioned earlier, this syndrome increases your risk of stroke, heart disease, and type 2 diabetes.

High Blood Pressure

Also known as hypertension, this condition refers to a state when your systolic blood pressure (usually above 140) is consistently higher than your diastolic blood pressure (usually about 90). How does being overweight increase your risk of hypertension? Generally, a larger body size will increase your blood pressure because your heart will have to work harder to send the necessary supply of blood to all cells. In addition, your excess body fats can damage your kidneys (which help your body regulate blood pressure). High blood pressure can result in kidney failure, heart diseases, and stroke.

Fatty Liver Disease

This is when there is a build-up of fat around the liver which can cause damage. If left unchecked, this damage can progress to liver failure.

Reproductive issues

Menstrual issues such as irregular menstrual cycles can occur in overweight women. Being overweight also increases the risk of infertility and complications during pregnancy.

Cancer

If you are obese or overweight, then the risk of developing cancer of the breast, gallbladder, colon, and endometrial lining of the uterus increases.

These are only some of the diseases associated with being overweight. Not to mention the social, emotional, and psychological impact of the extra weight.

WHY IT IS SO HARD TO LOSE WEIGHT

Being overweight, particularly if you have several pounds to lose as I did, isn't just unfortunate; it very well may be perilous. When I arrived at my highest weight of 450 pounds, I was informed that I was pre-diabetic and that if I were to proceed with my lifestyle, I would not be around for more than a couple more years. This scared me, and I realized the time had come to lock in, deal with myself, and lose the weight so I could stay with people around me.

This was more difficult than one might expect, in any case, and I realized that the road ahead would not be simple. I had attempted to get more fit before, and I bombed on numerous occasions. I didn't have a clue why I had fizzled out or how I planned to beat these disappointments to at long last lose the weight and keep it off for good.

If you've dieted previously, odds are this is a recognizable story. Before I could lose the weight, I needed to figure out why I had trailed off previously and what I could do to be fruitful later.

Defining Unrealistic Goals

When individuals start attempting to change the manner in which they eat, they set their objectives too high and attempt to immediately do a lot without any delay. Instead, as I began to get thinner, I started to construct my solid habits a little at a time. I gradually cut things like dairy and soft drinks out of my diet, as opposed to tossing everything out simultaneously.

When you attempt to accomplish overly ambitious objectives, for example, trying to change many habits at once in the short-term, then chances are you'll wind up feeling overwhelmed and unmotivated. Rather, attempt to find a way to eat better. For instance, rather than totally giving up soft drinks, pick a few soft drink options that you can switch out without much of a challenge.

Not Eating Nutritiously

A large number of individuals who attempt to get thinner commit the error of not eating adjusted, nourishing meals. When this occurs, the body responds, and you may get headaches, fatigue, feel overly moody, and crave specific—often unhealthy—foods. This can make you either abandon your fitness goals or go through periods of binge eating. If you need to get thinner, you can't simply zero in on calorie control. You additionally need to ensure that what you are eating is nutritious and your meals furnish your body with what it needs.

Crash Dieting

An endless number of individuals end up on crash diets to lose weight rapidly. This does not work in the long-term, particularly if you have a lot of weight to lose. It is not sustainable, so any weight lost on a crash diet will come back.

Not only does crash dieting not work, it can also be risky. Individuals who crash diet can experience symptoms like discomfort, irritability, fatigue, and cravings. Crash dieting can likewise slow your digestion, cause you to lose muscle, increase your risk of heart failure if done for a long time, weaken your immune system, and cause an unhealthy relationship with food.

Absence of Support

Getting thinner and adhering to your diet can be extremely challenging, particularly when there is nobody around you to support you, compliment you on your triumphs, and above all, be there when the challenges try to overpower you. Building an emotionally supportive network and encircling yourself with the perfect individuals can be the difference between progress and disappointment, so be certain you have a strong network. Where you find that help is up to you, regardless of whether it be your family, companions, or even online help.

Not Seeing Results Fast Enough

Getting in shape is intense because it requires some patience to see the results. Take crash dieting and weight loss pills which are so mainstream today, yet they don't work. Sure, they may seem to give you quick results, but weight loss isn't something that happens in a week or even a month. It requires significant investment, particularly when you do it the correct way, in order to see enduring weight loss results.

Negative Thoughts Can Affect Losing Weight

It appears everybody nowadays is attempting to lose weight. We are pressured by our peers and society to look, dress, and even act a specific way.

Each time you look at a magazine, turn on the TV, or see yourself in the mirror, you are reminded of society's ideals. You may hate your body for your lack of control, be disappointed in yourself, feel guilty and apprehensive, and now and again even feel discouraged.

The notion of shedding fat and losing weight seems simple at first glance. It is just eating fewer calories than your body requires and doing some activity to help your metabolism. But if it's that simple, why do so many people still struggle to lose weight?

You may realize that when you are feeling down or depressed, you tend to eat as a source of comfort. Generally, using food as a source of comfort or happiness isn't healthy and will turn into a deeply-ingrained habit; thus, whenever you experience any kind of stress or anguish, this triggers you to eat.

Struggling with negative thoughts about your life and yourself can hinder you from pushing ahead. You may have a habit of rewarding yourself for your successes with things that prevent you from losing weight. When you use food to reward or repay yourself, you may cause your progress to stall.

Although the struggles that I am alluding to around emotional eating are not healthy ones, they can likewise be utilized intentionally to get a specific outcome.

Emotional eating doesn't happen because you are physically hungry. It occurs because something triggers a craving for food or a specific nutrient. You are either subconsciously or deliberately denying yourself something that you need.

Similarly, the fear of eating can assume control over your life. It monopolizes your thoughts, depleting you of your vitality and self-discipline, until you lose yourself and binge eat. Eventually, it will cause more fear and make problems much worse.

So how might you conquer your fear and different feelings around eating?

You can transform the majority of your feelings around eating into another more beneficial relationship.

In all actuality, you have a soul. You can find it if you look. It is that spot inside of you that is continually thankful, forgiving, and tranquil. It speaks to your higher self, the genuine you, the sheltered, loved, and entire you. When you find this, the resentment, dissatisfaction, and stress that you are feeling about your weight will vanish.

Things often don't happen as rapidly as we might want them to. Maybe your body isn't changing as fast as you want it to. This may discourage you and give you further reason to indulge.

You must acknowledge and understand that your body is a gift, it's your temple! You have to begin to contemplate it.

Quit focusing on your stomach fat, your fat arms and butt, your enormous thighs that you hate, and every one of the calories that you're taking in, and see all that your body is, all that your body can do, and all that your body is doing...right now.

This new mindfulness will foster love for and understanding of your body like you've never had before. You'll start to treasure it like the astounding gift that it is and center yourself around fostering its well-being every day, in each moment, with each breath.

Begin concentrating on creating well-being as opposed to losing weight, and you will be increasingly happy, alive, and thankful. Find the delight of carrying on with a healthy life and feeding your soul consistently. Develop more love with your body and yourself, and this love will move and transform you from the inside out.

When you tap into something that is greater than you, you have constant motivation, which is far stronger than any battle of the mind or feelings. Accepting and adoring your body precisely as it is right now is what will send the healing vibrations that will quiet your mind and transform your body from the inside out.

When you figure out how to love and acknowledge your body, you are in-tune with your higher self, which is infinitely adoring and inviting.

Grasp what your identity is and not who you think you are or ought to be. Understand the endeavors that you make are like seeds. Try not to see the majority of your efforts to lose weight as disappointments, and instead consider them to be seeds you are planting towards progress.

Pardon yourself. Try not to beat yourself up, regardless of how frequently you think you've fizzled, irrespective of what you resemble at this moment and irrespective of how often you need that new beginning. Forgive yourself!

PART 2: BAD EATING HABITS

Bad eating habits are significant deviations of behavior that show themselves as eating patterns that are dangerous for your health. Bad eating habits have been on the rise since the COVID-19 pandemic hit. The most common types of bad eating habits are:

- Emotional Eating
- Binge Eating
- Mindless Eating

Emotional Eating

Emotional eating can best be defined as using eating as a means of coping with stress and difficult situations in life. This can become chronic, in order to fill in a void or gap in our life that we have challenges dealing with. In some cases, where this becomes a recurring and extreme, eating disorders may result.

For most people, it's a sign that we are responding to stress, grief, and other feelings with food, even when we do not experience hunger. This results in a pattern of binge-eating or overeating and in some cases, going without food until the hunger pangs become unbearable, causing us to overeat. In extreme cases, bulimia or anorexia are examples of eating disorders that cause us to avoid food (anorexia) or bounce between eating too much and forcing ourselves to eliminate food and lose weight (bulimia).

Food can represent more than nourishment. It is seen as a reward, a coping mechanism, or a comfort. The term "comfort food" signifies the need for food as a way to deal with a hardship, such as a relationship break up, losing a job, or a sense of failure when an expectation isn't met. It's counterproductive in the long-term, but it makes us feel good right away. Movies and television shows will sometimes show a character binging on a tub of ice cream after breaking up with their partner. This is an emotional response to a difficult experience.

Growing up, we learn to associate food with different aspects of our life. A lollipop or ice cream cone as a reward for good behavior or an extra slice of cake for helping with chores. It can also be restrictive, even punitive when portions or types of food are limited if we were pressured to lose weight and eat a certain way.

Both may have had positive intentions, but ultimately, we learn from childhood to see food as a tool to reward, punish, or comfort. It's not an easy pattern to reverse, though it can be done by acknowledging these traits that have been ingrained into us at a young age and recognizing the response to food when we experience one of these in adulthood:

- A reward as an adult may entail having an extra slice of cake to reward good eating habits during the first week of a diet.
- A punishment may be restricting what you eat over the next month to make up for or "correct" a binge or period of time when you ate foods considered forbidden when following a diet.
- Choosing to eat to cope with the grief of loss, stress, or frustration from occurrences in life.

What is the first sign of emotional eating? Cravings! These are common and we experience them daily. Cravings occur even when you are not hungry, as a response to an event. For example, if you feel stressed at work, you may crave chocolate or a bag of chips. The flavor may be appealing, as well as the texture or taste.

It may seem incidental at first to satisfy a craving with a small piece of chocolate, but because the response to stress is food-related, it will continue and become habit-forming. The initial sensation of tasting a piece of milk chocolate after handling a difficult client on the job may feel euphoric, and then you'll want another piece, followed by another. A pattern emerges that becomes a link between your emotions and food. The portions may also grow, as you soothe your woes, but in the end, there is no solution, and your eating habits become difficult to maintain.

How can you avoid the pitfalls of emotional eating? Take into consideration your mood when you reach for the next snack. Where are you currently? At work, home, at an event, or in a situation that causes a certain feeling? Most importantly, determine if you are actually hungry by using a scale from one to ten. If you rate your hunger closer to ten, it may be a good idea to eat, though make sure you find a calm place without stress before you begin your meal. Experiencing hunger means it's a good time to eat, but only with as little pressure and emotional impact as possible. If you are in a busy environment, find another space to decompress and relax. Practice deep breathing and decide where to enjoy your meal.

When you crave food, ask yourself what you are feeling. Are you angry, sad, or stressed? If you are experiencing an intense emotion or are in a state of frustration, hold off on eating until you can bring yourself into a calm space, away from any surroundings that are contributing to these emotions. It can take less time than you think and can be as easy as leaving the office or workspace and going outdoors to walk in a nearby park.

If that option is not available, choose a quiet place in your workplace with minimal distractions. Sometimes this can be difficult to find if your space is very busy and hectic. Even a few moments in a bathroom or an empty room for five minutes can make a big difference.

When you feel calmer, you may notice those cravings subside. It's okay if they don't, as stressful situations are not easy to diffuse. A few minutes can make the difference between reacting to your emotions with food and choosing another means to acknowledge and remedy the situation with meditation and a few moments of solitude.

Food is a good distraction. To identify your emotional connection to food means to acknowledge it mindfully, instead of making an excuse for it. It's common and easy to excuse eating simply to soothe a bad day or situation. Some emotions can be traced back to childhood or a significant experience that triggers a response with food. In these cases, it may take longer to delve deep within our minds to find the reason for the response.

Mindfulness helps us by taking a scan of our body and thoughts in that very moment and finding the root of that emotion. Are we feeling a quicker heartbeat or shallow breathing or something in our stomach? If someone upsets or insults you, food can quiet the injury temporarily, but it will only arise later when you realize that the source of conflict and emotion was not handled, but rather, avoided with food.

Binge Eating

Binge eating disorder is something that needs proper care, time, management, and treatment. Your whole lifestyle has to be turned upside down in order to be totally cured. There are many misconceptions regarding binge eating disorder. The first step to treating this disorder is to brush off all the myths.

You can treat binge eating disorder if you identify it and get proper help. If you are afraid of the consequences and how the people you know will react to this problem, it will only hamper you more. You need to counter your fears and get help as soon as you can. Dilly dallying will only make the problem worse.

We will go over many of the potential causes of binge eating disorder, but keep in mind that not every cause applies to everyone and not every tip will work for everyone. You'll need to seek treatment that is proportional to your struggles with the disorder.

Binge eating is as serious as any other mental health issue, and it should be treated carefully. Do not confuse it with overeating or bulimia. Take proper steps, work on your bad habits, and develop good habits over time.

The process will take some time, so be patient. Get help from your friends and family. You cannot do it alone. You need to get help from your loved ones and/or a professional.

Causes of Binge Eating Disorder

There are many potential causes of binge eating disorder. Research has been conducted to study this issue and several science-backed causes have been found. Unlike most diseases, there are no drug-based treatments available to cure binge eating disorder. No doctor on earth can write you a prescription to alleviate binge eating disorder. Instead, psychological and mental work will be needed. Right now, let us talk about the real causes behind binge eating disorder.

Biological

Although there is no single reason for every case of binge eating disorder, there are many causes, incidents, and situations in life that can trigger it. Some of the uncomplicated reasons are biological. When your family has a big history of binge eating disorder, then you are more likely to fall victim to binge eating disorder sooner or later. People can inherit this disorder genetically.

This sounds really crazy but it is true. Just like if your family has a history of a great metabolism, you are more likely to have a high metabolism yourself without trying hard with any diet. It can be a habit or genetic factor that comes from your father or mother. Growing up, if you noticed your parents or any sibling struggling with binge eating, then it is a cue for you to be extra cautious with food. Even if you do not have the problem yourself right now, it can come at any point in your life. So be prepared for it.

Not Eating Mindfully

One of the reasons behind binge eating disorder is that people eat emotionally and not mindfully. Eating emotionally is terrible for you as life does not always stay on track and bad incidents are very common. You cannot guarantee happiness even when you have all the materialistic things in life. Someone with an unlimited credit card can still be unhappy about life. People who tend to eat according to their mood develop a very bad eating habit. They may think to themselves that it is only a piece of candy, or a piece of cake, or an extra bite of the sandwich or an extra serving of rice, etc.

There are tons of examples where people try to convince themselves that the extra food they are consuming will not affect them. They can always exercise, eat less the next time, and it will all balance out. The truth of the matter is, it only leaves you one step closer to a bigger problem like bulimia or binge eating disorder. If you eat emotionally, you will find yourself struggling with food every time you feel depressed, every time you are feeling lonely, every time you go through a bad break up, every time you face failure, every time you do not achieve your goal, etc.

This eating emotionally and telling lies to yourself has to stop if you want to live a healthier life.

Loneliness

Being lonely is one of the biggest fears for almost everyone. There is no one on earth who would like to be alone. There are people who may say they enjoy their alone time. They may not be lying, but there are always a few loved ones who everyone wants to be around all the time. When their loved ones avoid them, they simply cannot take it. They cannot deal with that loneliness properly.

Today everyone is busy and you cannot talk or meet with your loved ones all the time. It is important that you let them have their space and support them without hurting the foundation of your relationship. This is not the case in romantic relationships only. People can get hurt and build a shield around them to block friends and family as well. This loneliness often triggers bad habits like emotional eating.

Often, emotional eating starts as an occasional indulgence. Then, faster than you can blink, it becomes a regular thing. Before you can spot it, it will turn into a binge eating disorder. So, you should learn to deal with loneliness in a healthy way. If you know you cannot handle loneliness, you need to take action to avoid being lonely. Make new friends, explore the city, try to be creative, and be the best version of yourself. You should not feel lonely even when you are alone. You should be able to enjoy your own company. Loneliness often triggers depression, and a depressed person is vulnerable to many mishaps.

Failure

Failure is devastating and you'd be hard-pressed to find someone who has not experienced failure in their life. Life is a roller coaster ride and there will be ups and downs. There is no standstill in this life. If one month is going well in your life, be prepared that the next month could be devastating. This is the circle of life, and dealing properly with failure is something you must learn to do.

People often deal negatively with failure. They cannot take the lesson that particular failure has taught them. They do not reflect on the failure, rather they try to get out of the phase of failure as soon as they can. This is not a healthy way to deal with failure. You always should reflect on your mistakes. Failure can come from many things. The smart way to deal with it is to learn from it. If you do not learn from it, you will end up making the same mistake again. People often use food as a shield to avoid their memories of failure. They start filling their stomach with food and think it will automatically erase their nasty failure feelings.

Food is never the solution. But the people who cannot deal with rejection and failure properly often take shelter in food. They eat as much as they can until they literally cannot remember the horrible memories of the failure. This is a very unhealthy way of dealing with failure as it does not really erase the memories, it only blocks them temporarily. But the horrible memories will come back soon to haunt you. On the other side, your body has to pay the price. Your body becomes lethargic, you start developing a bad sleeping routine and your skin becomes bad too. Most importantly you become obese and lazy. We will talk about the harmful effects binge eating disorder can have on your body and mind later.

False Body Image

Most of us no matter which region, which country we are living in, have a false notion of beauty. Beauty comes from within the heart, but most of us are not aware of the inner beauty that should be the talk of the town all the time. Inner beauty should be cherished for years, but inner beauty is something most of us are not even aware of. Inner beauty can never age, get wrinkles, or be ruined. It only gets better if you let it grow and blossom. We are so concerned about outer beauty all the time because it is there for everyone to see.

The media plays a very vital role here. Since our childhood, we have been taught to admire the people that had fair skin, nice long eyes, good thick eyebrows, a long thin nose, nice blonde hair, and blue eyes. Toni Morrison even wrote a novel on the false image of beauty, *The Bluest Eye*, where a kid is obsessed with having the bluest eye and fair skin, and her entire life revolves around trying to imitate what their society calls beautiful. She never obtains that beauty and ends up becoming a mental patient.

This is the case for most of us; we always try to attain that false beauty that has been stuck in our heads since childhood. We never consider the fact that the things we see are not always real. They are made to look good so that they can appeal to many people. They do it to sell their product and make money. But we never consider it unrealistic. We think if they can do it, so can you by maintaining a proper diet. To attain that unrealistic beauty, we often go out of our way. When after doing many things, we still cannot reach the goal, we tend to go the other way and build a bad eating habit. This bad eating habit soon becomes binge eating disorder.

This false image of beauty is not realistic and there is no one who would be able to achieve it without harming their own body. Many people who have tried to attain the false beauty portrayed by the media ended up being stuck with an eating disorder.

Consuming Too Much Alcohol

Consuming too much alcohol can also be deadly. Alcohol is bad for us. There are many types of research that show people who do not regularly drink alcohol are much healthier and more active. They tend to develop fewer diseases than people who drink alcohol daily.

Consuming too much alcohol can lead to bad eating habits. Your stomach is never fulfilled by food. You feel hungry all the time. You want to eat all the time, but you do not enjoy eating anything. It messes up your digestive system. You constantly want processed food and crave it all the time. You are not happy with real food. All you want to eat all day long is the processed snacks. Snacks are light in nature and they will not stay in the stomach for long. Therefore, you remain hungry all the time and you tend to eat more than you need.

People who drink too much alcohol often have bad eating habits, and these can build up to binge eating disorder over time.

Eating Too Fast

This may sound weird, but eating too fast can also be a reason behind binge eating. When you do not chew your food properly and scarf everything down in a rushed manner, your body tends to consume more food than you actually require. Your body takes about 20 minutes to message your brain that it is full or needs more food. So, when you chew slowly and give your body time to process the food you are eating, it slowly sends the message to your brain that you can stop eating now. Chewing your food is essential in order to develop a good digestive system. Chewing also helps you to eat the right amount of food by preventing you from overeating.

The people who eat too fast always eat more than they require. It is also hard on your digestive system, as it will have to work harder to break the food down into smaller bits if you don't chew it well. This uses more energy, therefore, you get hungry soon again. If you had chewed your food properly, your body would be satisfied with less food and would have kept you energized for a longer period of time.

So, eating too fast is not good. Try to chew every bite of food you consume. It will help stop your binge eating problems and develop a good digestion system.

Eating Processed Food

When you eat processed food, it may taste amazing and make you feel really good while eating it, but it leaves a very bad feeling later on. You do not feel satisfied with your stomach, you may get a bad gas problem, and it messes up your mood too. You feel very lethargic and hungry again soon.

Processed food is very easy to get addicted to. You simply cannot have enough of it. The added artificial flavors may be the trigger. It tastes so good and addictive you keep on eating it until your stomach says no. A burp is usually a sign of your body verbally saying it no longer needs food. But some of us even refuse to take that sign into an account and keep on eating until they finish all the food that is available. This is a very unhealthy approach towards food.

Even if you are not following any diet, too much-processed food should never be consumed. Even if you are at a healthy weight, even then too much-processed food is bad for you. People should not be eating in excess even when they are in perfect shape. Binge eating may not affect you now, but it can make you obese and lethargic over a period of time. Your metabolism can be good now, but if you continue to binge eat, it may get worse and cause you to gain excess weight suddenly.

Not Drinking Enough Water

You may wonder, how does drinking water relate to binge eating? It does on a very large scale! Experts, doctors, and nutritionists always advise their clients to drink lots of water because it plays a vital role in keeping us healthy. Staying hydrated is always mandatory in keeping us in good shape. Dehydration can cause many diseases. It makes you weak; it makes you lethargic and breathless. On the contrary, when you have enough water, you feel good and look good. Water contributes to digestion too.

Now the question is, how does it relate to binge eating? Whenever you get a craving, if you drink one glass of water, your craving will just vanish away for the next 30 minutes. If you don't believe me, try it out yourself. See if it works or not! People who do not drink enough water are always feeling hunger pangs. The food that they are consuming is not properly getting digested either because of not drinking enough water.

To make sure they stay hydrated, many people build the habit of drinking 8 glasses of water or more every day. If you have 3 large meals a day and get 1 or 2 healthy snacks, you do not need to eat otherwise. Between these 5 meals, if you feel a craving for anything, be it healthy or junk, drink a glass of water. It will help you forget about the craving. Many people have successfully lost significant amounts of weight just by building this habit of drinking water whenever they have cravings outside their 5 meals. Remember it will not happen in a day, you need to build this habit with time.

Not Getting Sufficient Sleep

Sleeping is very important for sound health. Have you ever noticed how everyone advises having a good night's sleep before a big exam, a big interview, or a long journey? Basically, anything important in life requires good focus and dedication. This focus and dedication will only come when your head is clear. Sleep is crucial in order to remain calm and focused.

Not getting enough sleep can trigger many mental problems and health problems. One of the problems it creates is binge eating. When you stay up at night, you will feel hunger pangs more frequently. You may eat even when your body does not require it. This creates a bad habit of binge eating and before you know it, you will discover yourself binge eating during the day as well.

Eating 2-3 hours before you go to sleep is advised by the doctors as it is easier to digest the food. But if you stay up late in the night and keep eating until you pass out, this damages your digestive system. Whenever you feel hungry after 9-10 p.m., drink a glass of water.

Mindless Eating

Mindless eating comes when you are not focused on or aware of the quantity of the food you intake or that you are eating in the first place. It often takes place with some other activity simultaneously going on. For example, you're watching TV and eating chips out of the bag and before you know it, there are no more chips. Or, you're sitting at work at your office desk while the bowl of chocolates next to you slowly depletes to three. Or maybe you feel guilty about wasting food, so you eat everything on your plate, even though you realized you were full a few moments ago.

Mindless eating can impact weight loss goals as it contributes to your calorie intake. These kinds of habits can happen to all of us, and they probably did at one point. Because we get busy and stressed, we start multitasking. We reach for food without really thinking about hunger, eat without really enjoying the fullness of taste, and getting a meal becomes almost like a chore.

BEGINNING STEPS TO TAKE

It is important to identify behaviors that lead to mindless eating. When you find yourself in that autopilot eating mode, become aware of this habit and try to notice what you are doing while you undertake mindless eating. These actions are usually something like watching TV, working on a project on a laptop, driving in the car, etc., but it is important to think about what else you could replace food with in these scenarios. For example, try crocheting or knitting in front of the TV, replace food with a warm cup of tea, or listen to some podcasts while driving.

We already talked about the weekly meal plan. Work out what you are going to make during the week, make a shopping list, and shop for the ingredients. This will help you stay organized and focused, it will save your budget as you won't buy any unnecessary food.

Incorporate movement into your daily life, we all know exercise is one of the crucial health components. Find time for a short walk or gentle stretching in the evening. Create mindful eating affirmations because they will help you in two ways. Firstly, with affirmations, you have a constant reminder of what is important to you, and secondly, they work to rewire your brain so that affirmation becomes second nature to you.

Get Off the Diet

Yes, we all want to lose that weight and we all think diets are the quickest way to achieve this goal. But the real goal is not losing weight in a short period and gaining it back again. The goal is to be in control. You have to learn how to be in control of your eating, and the unexpected answer here is to stop trying to be in control. Whenever we put restrictions on our food, for example, you forbid yourself from sweets, it will just create a bigger craving for that food. So, get off the diets and start seeing and making a mental notice of the quantity of food you eat daily. Deprivation doesn't work, and it doesn't do any good for your physical and mental health.

Dieting is stressful to the body. You are suddenly cutting out some ingredients and therefore messing with metabolic and biochemical reactions occurring in the body. Diets make you ignore all the signals your body is sending. Thus, it is more sustainable to make small changes over time, instead of suddenly following a strict diet.

PART 3: GOOD EATING HABITS

One of the most common goals is to eat and look healthier. And to stay fit and achieve your weight-loss goal, you have to break your bad eating habits. Below are the good eating habits you should start following instead to achieve your weight loss goal.

HEALTHY EATING HABITS

Eating Less

Regulate the amount of food that you consume on a daily basis. This habit may not be easy to start first, but it's a must. You may experience hunger pangs as your body may go through a withdrawal phase. But that won't be so hard to overcome if you carefully choose the kind of food to have. Choose natural foods that will not only fill your body with nutrients but also satisfy your cravings.

Consume Less Alcohol

If you are a regular alcohol drinker, you may need to limit your alcohol consumption. Alcohol has a lot of negative effects on your body. Avoid heavily consuming alcohol since it is also related to weight gain.

Eat More Fruits and Vegetables

Fruits and vegetables fortify your body and give you all the nutrients and vitamins that your body needs.

Exercise Regularly

Exercise doesn't have to be such a hard task, and it doesn't have to take much of your time. All you need is 10 to 30 minutes of exercise per day, maybe a walk in nature or workout at home. Exercising will also relieve your stress, which is a main cause of weight gain. Check Part 4 for the different workouts that you can do at home.

SMALL HABITS THAT HELP TO LOSE WEIGHT

Set Goals

When you set your goals, make sure that they are realistic and measurable. For instance, if you have two or more cups of coffee a day, challenge yourself to drink one cup of coffee and another cup of green tea. Make your goals clear and quantifiable. Don't tell yourself that you want to reduce your alcohol consumption; instead, tell yourself that you'll only have one drink once every two or three days.

Replace Coffee With Tea

Coffee is high in caffeine and in many cases, also rich in sugars. Make it a habit to substitute coffee for tea on a daily basis. Tea comes in different flavors, so you'll have a variety of choices that may suit your taste!

Add Cayenne Pepper to Your Dishes

Cayenne pepper has gained a lot of popularity in the West lately, but it's an ancient ingredient in many Indian, African, and Far Eastern dishes. If you are up for the spice, add cayenne pepper and other chili spices to your dishes. Mainly, it is the capsaicin in the chilies that burns fat faster.

Say No to Processed Fats

Believe me, it is the worst thing you could eat! Their only function is to add fat to your body. Instead, add lean protein to your diet. Lean meats don't only reduce weight, but they also satiate you better and boost your metabolism.

Cycle Your Carbs

We all love carbs, but we also know they are our worst enemy! Set it as a goal to cut down on carbs. You may even consider following a keto diet every once in a while.

Always Start With a Salad

Salads are a great way to start your meal. They are full of vitamins and nutrients. They will also satiate you and make you eat less.

Drink Water

Water is the panacea for all. Water fills you up. It is advisable to start your day with at least two cups of lukewarm water. Drink at least 2L of water a day to nourish and revitalize your body.

Weigh Yourself

Make it a habit to weigh yourself and keep a record of your weight. If you feel that your body weight is stuck, you may consider visiting a dietician to help you with a food plan.

Do Not Use Elevators

Consider it as a chance to exercise. Going up the stairs will vitalize your heart and lungs. Tighten your core and be mindful of your breathing the next time you take the stairs.

Do Not Go Grocery Shopping When Hungry

How often do we go grocery shopping and end up buying munchies and junk food that are just fatty? Before you do your grocery shopping, have a meal or at least a snack. Be mindful as you shop, and always look for healthier alternatives.

Steamed Veggies

Why not exchange fries or wedges with steamed veggies? This is a very important habit that you can develop which will definitely help you lose weight.

Avoid Frying

Baking is the alternative! I know nothing compares to crispy fried chicken, but you can easily swap out baking instead of frying. Add a few drops of oil and put your chicken in the oven. It will taste the same yet is way healthier.

Watch the Dressing

How often do you drop all the side dressing over your salad and end up with an extra moist salad? What you need to do is use a fork to dip in the dressing, and then use it to eat your salad. Often the ingredients in dressings include oils that are fatty so you shouldn't eat too much.

Start Your Day With Oats

Oats will energize you and satiate you in the morning. It's a great way to start your day. You may add yogurt, fruits, and nuts to the oats to make them tastier.

Share the Meal

Most of the time, the portions at restaurants are huge! A lot of times we also want to try more than one item. Why not share your meal with someone, that way you'll have a smaller portion, and you may also share a salad or an appetizer.

Avoid the Dessert

How many times have you finished a big meal and forgot to leave a space for dessert, yet you have one? What I usually do is save the dessert at dinner, that's if I don't want to exceed my calories per day.

Walk and Not Drive

If you have certain errands that you can do while walking instead of driving, do so! I usually make a list of my daily errands and often end up doing several errands in one walking trip. Whether it's rainy or sunny, it's always fun to take a walk.

Order From Healthy Joints

Forget about ordering pizza or burgers. There are many other alternatives. Check the places near you that deliver healthy meals. Save these to your contacts. There are many restaurants that deliver healthy and tasty meals.

Laugh, Laugh, and Laugh Again!

Believe it or not, laughter helps you burn calories. I know it's not much, but laughter also makes you more positive and releases your stress, hence helping your body stabilize and lose weight.

Avoid Socializing Around Meals Too Much

You don't have to eat to socialize. Accept invitations when you know that there will only be healthy food, such as a grill or barbeque, and avoid those with pizza and alcohol. This will not only help you, but it will encourage your friends to do the same as well.

Replace Junk With Healthy Snacks

Your cravings for salty or sugary, fatty snacks will fade away once you avoid them for a few days. When you feel like having a snack, have some nuts or dried fruits. Bake some oat cookies and add some raisins to them. These are healthy and will also strengthen your body.

Do Not Define Yourself Through Your Losses

Do not define yourself based on your losses. If you don't find yourself losing weight as fast as you expect, do not give up. Explore your body and keep records of the foods that you think help you lose weight and those that don't. Losing weight requires patience and determination, it won't happen overnight. If you find yourself falling off the wagon, get back on it. Make your expectations realistic so you won't fall into disappointment.

HABITS WORKBOOK

Acquiring and maintaining good habits is more feasible if you keep a record of your progress.

Readiness

Reflect on your weight loss journey. Think of what has worked for you and what challenges you have faced. It's always good to look back at mistakes and experiences and learn from them.

Use the table below to aid you with this. Take your time, the most important thing is to be honest with yourself.

Benefits	Challenges
Example: My body will be strong and energized.	Example: I'm not a big fan of exercising.

How Ready Are You to Start Your Weight Loss Journey?

This section will allow you to reflect on and evaluate your response to your past weight loss attempts. You may have tried different kinds of diets that didn't work, you may have lost weight but then quickly regained it, or you may have started a certain habit but then changed it. What changed? What made you shift your habits?

This table will help you:

1. Identify the habits or plans that worked and helped you. What did you do right in your previous weight loss attempts?
2. List the challenges you have faced. Why did you give up or shift your habits? What new habits did you acquire? What made you change your mind?

Previous Weight Loss Attempts	
What went right? What worked well?	What challenges did you face? What didn't you like about the attempt?

Lifestyle

As mentioned before, you have to make some alterations to your lifestyle. It is important to also keep a record of the habits that you feel you should incorporate in your life and the benefits you will gain from them. Assess how you will approach these habits and what will make you stick to them. The table below is to record your solutions. Before filling the table with your ideas, make sure to keep the following in mind:

- The amount of food you consume.
- What foods to buy.
- What better food alternatives do you have? Which ones do you like?
- Will you be cooking?
- Will alcohol be part of your new habits?
- What activities or exercises will you include in your daily routine, how do you plan to work on them, and how frequently?
- How will you deal with cravings?
- What prevents you from being active?

Challenges	Solutions

Activities

Keep track of the food you eat as well as your physical activities. If you skip an exercise, write down why you skipped it. For instance, write that you had many deadlines and couldn't afford even 10 minutes for a workout. This isn't meant to make you feel guilty, but to write down the obstacles that you face in order to find solutions for them.

The goal behind this is to transform you both physically and mentally into a better version of yourself. To keep the progress going, we will take it one step at a time.

Date and Time	Food and Drink Write down the chosen food, how you will cook it, and what portion size you had.	Notes How was the eating experience?	Activity Type What exercise did you do? For how long?

Goals

The SMART method is perfect to help you prepare and set your goals.

S is for Specific

If your goals are unclear, it will hinder your focus and efforts to achieve anything. Make your goals clear and specific.

M is for Measurable

Measuring your goals will help you calculate your progress or how far you have deviated away from your goals.

A is for Achievable

It doesn't mean not to be ambitious, but to set goals that are realistic. For example, telling yourself that you want to lose 20 kgs a month is far-fetched. Ask yourself, will you be able to achieve this goal? How hard will it be? What will you give up? Being too optimistic can lead to disappointment if what you are expecting isn't achievable.

R is for Relevant

If your goal is something like "I am only going to use natural ingredients and cook so that in two months I can write a book about it and be a master chef," then you might have to reconsider if this truly applies to you right now.

Make your goals relevant to your present situation. Tackle one goal at a time. Once you see yourself losing weight, maybe you can write a book and share your experience.

T is for Time-bound

Every goal that you create must have a target date. It's easy to tell yourself that you want to lose a certain amount of weight, but set a time span for it. How much will you lose in the coming two weeks or a month? That's better!

Check the following table which will help you prepare and set your goals.

My Goal	Example: To prepare healthy meals to eat at work.
Date Started	
S (Specific)	Example: Prepare a salad with nuts for lunch at work.
M (Measurable)	Example: I will prepare 5 meals, one for every day at work.
A (Achievable)	Example: I may not have time to prepare my meals in the morning, but I could prepare them in the evening before going to sleep.
R (Realistic)	Example: I have enough time at work during my lunch break to have my meal.
T (Time-bound)	Example: I want to make this a habit within the next two months.

Weight

When you set your weight-loss goals, divide them into feasible chunks. For example, take 5% of your current weight and then write a new target weight once you achieve the current one. Let your goal be to lose weight steadily, perhaps about a pound (0.5 kgs) per week. This is achievable, but you can also aim for more.

Keep in mind to weigh yourself in the morning on a daily basis or once a week. Don't panic if your weight fluctuates, that's perfectly normal. Find your result at the end of the week and keep track of it.

Weight Target

Start Date	Target Weight	Target Achieve Date

Weight Tracker

Date	Weight	Change in Weight

PART 4: WORKOUTS

The most popular excuse for not working out is not having enough time, but you have to make the time. Working out for at least 10 minutes a day can benefit you a lot. It will help with blood flow, hormonal balance, and weight loss. The workouts in this part do not require any equipment and won't take much of your time, but they definitely show results. Exercising in the morning before you have your breakfast stimulates your body to burn more calories because you're already in the fat-burning stage before you eat.

The 30-Day Challenge

Make it your goal to commit to this 30-day workout challenge. This goal is SMART. You can control the duration of the workouts to suit your daily schedule. You may start with 10-minute intense workouts and then gradually increase the duration every one or two days.

It's important to vary your workouts every day. Target different parts of your body. This way exercising won't be boring. You may substitute these workouts with an outdoor jog or hike, or maybe even play basketball or football.

Push-Ups

To make push-ups fun and exciting, I take a couple of minutes as I'm doing my daily tasks to drop down and do 12 pushups. You don't have to start with a lot, try doing five today and ten tomorrow. If you need a more challenging variation, try the diamond push-up for a change. To do this, face the floor, stretch your feet out behind you, and press yourself up on the balls of your feet. In a triangle position, place both arms and make sure that your hands are under your chin, and form a diamond shape with your index fingers and your thumbs touching. Push yourself up from the floor. The diamond push-up is a little harder, so you should make sure you're comfortable with regular push-ups before trying it out. The most important thing is not to strain yourself.

Mountain Climber

In your first week of exercising, include ten mountain climbers daily. Whether it's a staircase or a flat floor, press on the balls of your feet as you support yourself on your hands. Then, mimic the movements of a mountain climber against the floor as you bring your knees closer to your torso.

Bicycle Crunching

Bicycle crunches are an amazing workout for your obliques, hips, and abs. Lie flat on your back, place your hands behind your head, slightly bend your knees, and then crunch your body. Get your left elbow as close as possible to your right knee, and then follow by the right elbow touching the left knee. Aim for twenty bicycle crunches a day!

Planks

Planks are fun and easy, and they burn fats around the stomach region. Challenge yourself with one 60-second plank a day to see good results. To ensure you have the right technique, rest your upper body on your forearms against the floor and elevate your lower body onto the balls of your feet. Make sure to straighten your spine and hold your entire body in a straight line.

Jumping Squats

Squats are fun and easy, especially as we await the booty outcome. But jumping squats are fun and challenging. Jumping squats get your triceps, calves, and buttocks working. First, stand with your legs shoulder-width apart, straighten your arms, bend your knees gently, and let the shoulders come forward as you extend your arms in front of you. Release the position as you jump when you reach the top. You may lose your balance in your first attempts, but don't give up. Do three repetitions of 10 jumping squats a day.

Cycling or Rowing

These are fun workouts that will require you to buy the equipment if you don't regularly go to the gym. Cycling and rowing are great cardiovascular workouts that give the entire body a flex. Cycling or rowing for ten minutes a day can be an effective part of your 30-day challenge.

10-MINUTE WORKOUTS

It sounds encouraging to have workouts that take only 10 minutes. These you can easily do in your mornings before going to work. You will start your day with a boost of energy. These workouts specifically target certain areas of your body.

Beginner's Choice

This is the perfect way to start your exercise and weight loss journey, and it can easily be added to your 30-day challenge. This exercise works your abs. Every round of exercise should be for 30 seconds, and then take another 30 seconds to rest.

Start out by lying flat on your back and bending your knees. Support your head using the palms of your hands. Then start doing middle crunches as you raise your shoulders.

Rest for 30 seconds.

Then, turn onto your left side and bend your knees into the same position as the middle crunch. Pull your shoulders forward using force with your hands as you place them behind your head. Move your torso and left elbow towards your highest knee.

Rest for 30 seconds.

Now, turn to the right and bend your knees into the same position as the previous exercise. Crunch to the right now and bring your right elbow as close as you can to the top knee.

Rest for 30 seconds.

Lie down on your back and bend your knees. Use your core to lift your shoulder up off the ground so your hand slides along the ground to touch your heel. Alternate back and forth between each hand.

Rest for 30 seconds.

Lie on your back with your legs straight and then raise them as high as you can. Hold your arms straight against your sides. Hold your position for 10 seconds and repeat 3 times.

Rest for 30 seconds.

Sit and gently bend your knees. Hold your hands together in your lap and make sure your heels are touching the ground.

Then, gently lean backward and twist your hands to the left and right.

Rest for 30 seconds.

Go back to your seated position, lean your shoulders backward, and slightly bend your knees. Cross your arms over your chest and hold this position.

Rest for 30 seconds.

Take the mountain climbing position. Raise your knee close to your upper body, then alternate between raising each knee.

Rest for 30 seconds.

Do a plank and hold it. Remember to keep your back and legs straight in a line.

Rest for 30 seconds.

Lie down on your back and raise your legs straight. Stretch your arms toward your feet like the toe touch exercise.

Rest for 30 seconds.

Now is the time for bicycle crunches. Lift your right leg off the ground and point it straight out. Your left leg should be lifted but bent at the knee. Use your abs to pull up into a crunch and touch your right elbow to your left knee. Switch leg positions and touch your left elbow to your right knee.

Rest for 30 seconds.

Bicycle Crunch

Start by doing a hip lift, and remain on your back and raise your legs. Use the force in your arms for support and push your legs even higher. Drop them and repeat to push them up again, and never lose the support of your arms. You may swing your legs back and forth to make it more effective.

Rest for 30 seconds.

Raise your legs again, and stretch your arms out straight along your sides. Hold this position. This is an ab hold which strengthens your core, arms, and thighs.

Rest for 30 seconds.

Next, do a spider plank and support yourself on your hands and the balls of your feet. Bring your left foot to your calf to form a triangle and then you can bring it back down. Alternate to the right leg and repeat the same position.

Rest for 30 seconds.

It's a great way to finish your ten-minute ab workout with another 60 second plank. Remember to keep your legs straight in a straight line with your back and support yourself on your forearms.

This was a great ab workout. You can add it to your 30-days challenge and track the changes that you see in your body.

Belly-Burner

This workout is low-impact and will strengthen your full-body. It targets belly fat and the legs. This time, the exercises will be for thirty seconds while the rest period is for 10 seconds.

Start by going into a knee pull as you scissor your legs and face a 45-degree angle. Lift your arms up above your head and then bring them down while you raise your back leg upward to meet your hands.

Rest for 10 seconds.

Alternate sides and do knee pulls on the other leg.

Rest for 10 seconds.

Stand and place your hands in front of your face as if you're praying, and then lean towards your left side. Bend your left knee to support your body and keep your right leg straight. Bring the support knee back and shift your support to the right leg and let the left leg step behind the right one. Swing backward while you open your hands.

Rest for 10 seconds.

Repeat the earlier exercise using your right leg now.

Rest for 10 seconds.

Get down on your knees and clasp your hands in front of you. Use one leg at a time and get up from your knees and then use one leg at a time to go back down onto your knees.

Rest for 10 seconds.

Do the superman plank. Raise your left leg and right arm to straighten them. Try to keep your balance as you bring them back in and then alternate to the right leg and left arm.

Rest for 10 seconds.

This exercise is a squat front kick. Start by separating your legs shoulder-width apart and drop down with your hands in front of you. Let your shoulders come slightly forward and then give a kick forward as you rise again.

Rest for 10 seconds.

Next, is the crab squat. To get into this position, start with the squat position. Squat down, and come up. Step in with one leg and out with the other to "crab walk" sideways. Alternate directions as you work.

Rest for 10 seconds.

Go down and do a push-up and then stand up back again. Step back, step forward, and then do another push-up. Repeat for 30 seconds.

Rest for 10 seconds.

Do mountain climbers for 30 seconds. Make sure to bring your knees as close as you can to your upper body with each step.

Rest for 10 seconds.

Take the side plank position. Rest yourself on your left forearm, facing towards the wall. Rest your legs on the side of your left foot. Lift your right hand up over your shoulder and then bring it back.

Rest for 10 seconds.

Shift to a side plank position on your right side now. Lift your left arm up above your shoulder and then bring it back down.

Rest for 10 seconds.

This exercise is corkscrews. To do this, go into the push-up position and then bring your left leg under your core. Kick it out toward your right side and touch it with your right hand. Return to the starting position and switch to the other leg and hand. You may lose your balance the first couple of times, but soon you'll be able to maintain your balance.

Rest for 10 seconds.

Sit down and rest your upper body on your hands placed flat on the ground close behind you. Then, raise your legs as you kick them forward while your upper body gently moves back.

Rest for 10 seconds.

Take the table position and then raise your core as high as you can. Rest your hands and feet on the ground to make a table shape. Rise and drop your core for 30 seconds.

Rest for 10 seconds.

Position yourself in the traditional push-up stance to do a shoulder tap. Lift your left hand to tap your right shoulder and then drop it. Then, alternate to the right hand and left shoulder.

Rest for 10 seconds.

You're almost done. Now is the time to do reverse lunges. Start by standing straight and scissoring your left leg backward and bend your right knee. Bring your hands up to meet in front of you, and then bring your leg back. Switch to the other leg and repeat the lunge as before.

Rest for 10 seconds.

Finally, it's the forward lunge. Stand with your feet shoulder-width apart. Hold a dumbbell in each hand. Make sure to start with the dumbbell weight that suits you. Take a long stride forward with your right leg and then lower into a lunge. Bend your knees and keep your posture upright. Make sure your knees do not go over your toes. Lean towards your front heel and return to a standing position.

Switch legs and repeat.

Congratulations! You have completed another workout! Make sure to drink plenty of water and do some stretching.

Yoga

Yoga has been shown to benefit many and help them lose weight in a healthy way. Yoga, along with a healthy diet, has proven to help in losing weight as well as supporting your mind and body. Yoga teaches you to be mindful and to relate better to your body. Yoga will also encourage you to maintain a healthy diet as it helps you develop a positive mindset.

Yoga does not only help you shed the fat, but it also has the following benefits:

- Stress management
- Better flexibility
- Improved breathing
- Boosts energy and vitality
- Balanced metabolism
- Muscle toning
- Enhances cardiovascular health
- Weight loss

Stress is the main cause of many of our physical and mental health problems. That's why yoga is so useful, as it helps you to manage your stress and give you physical exercise, which will lead you to lose weight and maintain physical and mental strength.

Best Yoga Poses for Weight Loss

- Sun salutation does not only warm up the muscles and get the blood flowing, but it also stretches and tones your muscles, waist, and arms. It also boosts your metabolism.
- Wind releasing pose helps you drop the extra fat on your stomach area.
- Intense side stretch pose benefits in burning calories and in reducing fat from your sides.
- Bow pose helps you in dropping the excess fat from the arms and legs and gaining muscle tone.
- Eagle pose helps in making your thighs, legs, and arms thinner.
- One-legged downward-facing dog tones your arms, abdominal muscles, thighs, and legs.
- Cobra pose is helpful in firming buttocks and in toning abdominal muscles.
- Plank pose strengthens your core and abdominal muscles.
- Warrior pose tones your thighs, shoulders, back ends, legs, and arms. And guess what? It'll help you gain that coveted flat stomach!
- Triangle pose improves digestion and reduces belly and waist fat.
- Downward dog pose tones your whole body and strengthens your arms, thighs, hamstrings, and back.
- Shoulder stand boosts overall strength, improves digestion, improves metabolism, and balances thyroid levels.
- Bridge pose is perfect for glutes. It tones and strengthens muscles, improves digestion, and balances hormones thyroid levels.
- Corpse pose is a very important pose to end your workout session as it helps your muscles relax to avoid muscle injury.

PART 5: HEALTHY RECIPES

Let's admit it, we all love food! Food isn't just essential for our survival, but also something that we like and enjoy. Too bad that the foods we tend to crave are not very healthy, but it's quite easy to make some substitution in the ingredients to prepare a healthy and delicious meal. The recipes in this part are easy to make, and most ingredients can be found in your local supermarkets. Don't forget to try to snack recipes, they will blow your mind!

BREAKFAST RECIPES

Smoked Salmon Omelette

Preparation time: 45 minutes

Cooking time: 15 minutes

Servings: 2

Ingredients:

- 2 medium eggs
- 3.5 ounces smoked salmon, cut
- 1/2 teaspoon capers
- 1 pinch (0.3 ounces) rocket, diced
- 1 teaspoon parsley, diced
- 1 teaspoon extra virgin olive oil

Directions:

1. In a bowl, whisk the eggs well.
2. Add in the salmon, capers, rocket, and parsley.
3. Warm up the olive oil in a nonstick skillet until hot yet not smoking.
4. Add in the egg blend and use a spatula to move the mixture around the dish until it is even.
5. Turn down the heat and let the omelet cook through.
6. Slide the spatula around the edges and move up or crease the omelet to fold in half and serve.

<u>*Date and Walnut Porridge*</u>

Preparation time: 55 minutes

Cooking time: 30 minutes

Servings: 2

Ingredients:

- 7 ounces milk (optional)
- 1 medjool date, chopped
- 1 ounce buckwheat chips
- 1 teaspoon pecan spread or four cleaved pecans
- 2 ounces strawberries, hulled

Directions:

1. Heat milk while whisking.
2. Add buckwheat chips and cook until the porridge is your ideal consistency.
3. Mix in the pecan margarine or pecans, top with the strawberries, and serve.

Avocado Eggs With Toast

Preparation time: 10 minutes

Cooking time: 45 minutes

Servings: 2

Ingredients:

- 1 avocado
- 4 slices of bread
- 2 tablespoons avocado oil
- 4 medium eggs
- ½ teaspoon salt, separated into four portions
- ½ teaspoon ground pepper, separated into four portions
- 4 tablespoons salsa

Directions:

1. Preheat the oven to 375ºF. Use cooking spray to coat a large rimmed baking sheet.
2. Cut the avocado in half and strip. Cut the long way into 1/4-inch-thick cuts, so you have cut through the entire length of the avocado with the gap from the pit. Separate the four cuts nearest to either side of the hole and the external cuts. Set aside.
3. Use a baked good brush to delicately cover the two sides of each cut of bread with oil. Cut a piece out of the middle of each slice of bread so it looks like one of the external avocado slices.
4. Store the cut out pieces of bread, and transfer the bread with avocado-shaped holes to the readied baking sheet.
5. Add the avocado cuts in the gaps of the bread.
6. Split an egg over each of the avocado cuts in the bread. Sprinkle the eggs with ⅛ teaspoon salt and ⅛ teaspoon pepper. Place the remaining avocado slices from near the pit on top of the eggs.

7. Bake until the toast has seared in spots and the eggs have set, 10 to 12 minutes.
8. Top with salsa as you desire. Present with the cut-out bread pieces.

Chocolate Granola

Preparation time: 10 minutes

Cooking time: 38 minutes

Servings: 8

Ingredients:

- ¼ cup cacao powder
- ¼ cup maple syrup
- 2 tablespoons coconut oil, melted
- ½ teaspoon vanilla extract
- ⅛ teaspoon salt
- 2 cups gluten-free rolled oats
- ¼ cup unsweetened coconut flakes
- 2 tablespoons chia seeds
- 2 tablespoons unsweetened dark chocolate, chopped finely

Directions:

1. Preheat your oven to 300ºF and line a medium baking sheet with parchment paper.
2. In a medium pan, add the cacao powder, maple syrup, coconut oil, vanilla extract, and salt, and mix well.
3. Place the pan over medium heat and cook for about 2 to 3 minutes, or until thick and syrupy, stirring continuously.
4. Remove from the heat and set aside.
5. In a large bowl, add the oats, coconut, and chia seeds, and mix well.
6. Add the syrup mixture and mix until well combined.
7. Transfer the granola mixture into a prepared baking sheet and spread in an even layer.
8. Bake for about 35 minutes.
9. Remove from the oven and set aside for about 1 hour.
10. Add the chocolate pieces and stir to combine.

11. Serve immediately.

Blueberry Muffins

Preparation time: 15 minutes

Cooking time: 20 minutes

Servings: 8

Ingredients:

- 1 cup buckwheat flour
- 1½ teaspoons baking powder
- ¼ teaspoon sea salt
- 2 eggs
- ½ cup unsweetened almond milk
- 2 – 3 tablespoons maple syrup
- 2 tablespoons coconut oil, melted
- 1 cup fresh blueberries

Directions:

1. Preheat the oven to 350ºF and line 8 cups of a muffin tin.
2. In a separate bowl, place the eggs, almond milk, maple syrup, and coconut oil, and beat until well combined.
3. Now, add the flour mixture and continue mixing until just combined.
4. Fold the blueberries in gently.
5. Bake for about 25 minutes.
6. Remove the muffin tin from the oven and place it onto a wire rack to cool for about 10 minutes.
7. Carefully tip the muffins out onto a wire rack and let cool completely before serving.

Chocolate Waffles

Preparation time: 15 minutes

Cooking time: 24 minutes

Servings: 8

Ingredients:

- 2 cups unsweetened almond milk
- 1 tablespoon fresh lemon juice
- 1 cup buckwheat flour
- ½ cup cacao powder
- ¼ cup flaxseed meal
- 1 teaspoon baking soda
- 1 teaspoon baking powder
- ¼ teaspoons kosher salt
- 2 large eggs
- ½ cup coconut oil, melted
- ¼ cup dark brown sugar
- 2 teaspoons vanilla extract
- 2 ounces unsweetened dark chocolate, chopped roughly

Directions:

1. In a bowl, add the almond milk and lemon juice and mix well.
2. Set aside for about 10 minutes.
3. In a bowl, place buckwheat flour, cacao powder, flaxseed meal, baking soda, baking powder, and salt, and mix well.
4. In the bowl with the almond milk mixture, place the eggs, coconut oil, brown sugar, and vanilla extract, and beat until smooth.
5. Now, add in the flour mixture and mix until smooth.
6. Gently fold in the chocolate pieces.
7. Preheat the waffle iron and then grease it.
8. Place the desired amount of the mixture into the pre-

heated waffle iron and cook for about 3 minutes, or until golden brown.

9. Repeat with the remaining mixture.

Salmon and Kale Omelet

Preparation time: 10 minutes

Cooking time: 7 minutes

Servings: 4

Ingredients:

- 6 eggs
- 2 tablespoons unsweetened almond milk
- Salt and ground black pepper, to taste
- 2 tablespoons olive oil
- 4 ounces smoked salmon, cut into bite-sized chunks
- 2 cups of fresh kale, tough ribs removed and chopped finely
- 4 scallions, chopped finely

Directions:

1. In a bowl, place the eggs, coconut milk, salt, and black pepper, and beat well. Set aside.
2. In a non-stick wok or skillet, heat the oil over medium heat.
3. Add in and spread the egg mixture evenly and cook for about 30 seconds, without stirring.
4. Place the salmon, kale, and scallions on top of egg mixture evenly.
5. Now, reduce heat to low.
6. Cover the wok or skillet with a lid and cook for about 4 – 5 minutes, or until the omelet is done completely.
7. Uncover and cook for about 1 minute. Fold in half if desired.
8. Carefully, transfer the omelet onto a serving plate and serve.

Moroccan Spiced Eggs

Preparation time: 1 hour

Cooking time: 50 minutes

Servings: 2

Ingredients:

- 1 teaspoon olive oil
- 1 shallot, stripped and chopped finely
- 1 red bell pepper, deseeded and chopped finely
- 1 garlic clove, stripped and chopped finely
- 1 courgette (zucchini), stripped and chopped finely
- 1 tablespoon tomato puree
- ½ teaspoon stew powder or seasoning mix, as desired
- ¼ teaspoon ground cinnamon
- ¼ teaspoon ground cumin
- ½ teaspoon salt
- 400g (14oz) can peeled and chopped tomatoes
- 400g (14oz) may chickpeas in water
- A little bunch of level leaf parsley (10g (1/3oz)), diced roughly
- Four medium eggs at room temperature

Directions:

1. Heat the oil in a pan, add in the shallot and red pepper, and fry delicately for 5 minutes.
2. Add in the garlic and courgette (zucchini) and cook for another minute or two.
3. Add the tomato puree, seasonings and spices, and salt and mix through.
4. Add the chopped tomatoes and chickpeas on medium heat.
5. Cover the dish with a lid, allow the sauce to simmer for 30 minutes – ensure it is delicately bubbling all through and permit it to lessen in volume by around

30%.

6. Remove from the warmth and mix in the diced parsley.
7. Preheat the oven 350ºF.
8. When you are prepared to cook the eggs, bring the tomato sauce up to a delicate boil and move to a small broiler dish.
9. Crack the eggs on the dish and lower them delicately into the stew. Spread equally and bake in the oven for 10 - 15 minutes.
10. Serve the blend in separate dishes with the eggs sitting on the top.

Chilaquiles With Gochujang

Preparation time: 30 minutes

Cooking time: 20 minutes

Servings: 2

Ingredients:

- 1 dried ancho chili
- 2 cups of water
- 1 cup squashed tomatoes
- 2 cloves of garlic
- 1 teaspoon sea salt
- ½ tablespoons gochujang
- 5 to 6 cups of tortilla chips
- 3 large eggs
- 1 tablespoon olive oil
- Optional toppings: diced cilantro, cotija crumbles, spicy peppers, avocado slices, chopped onions

Directions:

1. Heat water in a pot till boiling
2. Add the ancho chile to the boiling water and cook for 15 minutes.
3. When completed, use a spoon to extricate the chili. Leave some of the water to prepare the sauce.
4. In a blender or food processor, process the boiled chili, 1 cup of saved boiled water, squashed tomatoes, garlic, salt, and gochujang until smooth.
5. Pour sauce into a large dish and place over medium heat for 4 to 5 minutes.
6. Lower the heat and add the tortilla chips. Mix the chips to cover with the sauce.
7. In another skillet, sprinkle a teaspoon of oil and fry an egg on top, until the whites have settled. Plate the egg and cook the remainder of the eggs.

8. Sear the eggs while you heat the red sauce.
9. Add the seared eggs and toppings of your choice over the chips.
10. Serve right away.

Baked Breakfast Potatoes

Preparation time: 1 hour, 10 minutes

Cooking time: 1 hour

Servings: 2

Ingredients:

- 2 medium reddish-brown potatoes, cleaned and pricked with a fork
- 2 tablespoons unsalted butter spread
- 3 tablespoons fresh cream
- 4 rashers cooked bacon
- 4 large eggs
- ½ cup shredded cheddar
- Evenly cut chives
- Salt and pepper to taste

Directions:

1. Preheat the oven to 400°F.
2. Place potatoes right on the grill rack for 30 to 45 minutes, flipping halfway.
3. Take out the potatoes and let cool for 15 minutes.
4. Cut every potato down the middle longwise and burrow each half out, scooping the potato into a blending bowl.
5. Mix butter and cream with the potato and knead until smooth—season with salt and pepper and mix.
6. Spread a portion of the potato blend into the base of each emptied potato skin and sprinkle with one tablespoon cheddar (you may keep the remaining mashed potato for a snack or other recipe).
7. Add one rasher of bacon to each half and top with a raw egg.
8. Place potatoes onto a greased or non-stick baking sheet.

9. Lower the oven temperature to 375 °F and heat potatoes until egg whites are lightly set and yolks are still runny.

10. Top every potato with a sprinkle of the rest of the cheddar, season with salt and pepper, and finish with cut chives.

Beef Stroganoff French Bread Toast

Preparation time: 10 minutes

Cooking time: 15 minutes

Servings: 2

Ingredients:

- 4 tablespoons olive oil
- ½ cups mushrooms
- 2 teaspoons salt, separated
- ½ teaspoon dark pepper
- 2 tablespoons thyme
- 2 tablespoons butter
- ½ cup onions, diced
- 2 cloves garlic, minced
- 1 pound ground meat
- 3 tablespoons of all purpose flour
- 2 teaspoons paprika
- ½ cups meat broth
- ½ cup sour cream
- 1 teaspoon Dijon mustard

For the toast:

- 1 portion French bread, inner parts dug out
- 2 cups mozzarella cheese
- 3 tablespoons cleaved Italian parsley

Directions:

1. Preheat the oven to 350°F, and line a baking sheet with parchment paper.
2. In a large Dutch grill or skillet, heat olive oil over medium heat.
3. Saute mushrooms with one teaspoon salt and dark pepper. Include thyme.
4. Cook mushrooms until tender, roughly for 4 minutes.

Remove from the skillet and set aside.

5. Add butter, onions, and garlic in the pot and saute for 2 minutes.
6. Cook ground meat over medium heat until it changes color, roughly 4 minutes.
7. Add flour and paprika to equally cover.
8. Add meat broth, sour cream, and Dijon mustard. Blend entirely and then add cooked mushrooms and top with mozzarella cheddar.
9. Place on the readied baking sheet, and bake for 5 to 10 minutes until cheddar is melted.
10. Sprinkle with parsley, cut, and serve right away.

Classic French Toast

Preparation time: 10 minutes

Cooking time: 45 minutes

Servings: 2

Ingredients:

- Four large eggs
- ½ cup low fat milk
- 1 teaspoon vanilla concentrate
- ½ teaspoons ground cinnamon partitioned
- 8 slices Brioche bread
- Optional toppings: maple syrup, powdered sugar, berries

Directions:

1. Preheat the frying pan to 350ºF.
2. Soften a little butter on the hot frying pan or in a large skillet over medium heat.
3. Add eggs and whisk well.
4. Mix in milk and a teaspoon of vanilla concentrate.
5. Dip each side of the bread in the egg blend. Note: Add the other portion of the cinnamon after you have coated half of your bread cuts and blend once more. This will ensure the bread slices get an equal measure of cinnamon on both sides.
6. Serve the French toast warm with maple syrup, powdered sugar, and berries, as desired.

Note: To keep the French toast warm, heat the stove to 200ºF. Place a wire rack on a large baking sheet and place the French toast on the shelf. Keep warm in the oven for as long as 30 minutes.

Avocado and Kale Omelet

Preparation time: 10 minutes

Cooking time: 45 minutes

Servings: 2

Ingredients:

- 2 large eggs
- 1 teaspoon low-fat milk
- ½ teaspoon of salt
- 2 teaspoons extra-virgin olive oil
- 1 cup cleaved kale
- 1 tablespoon lime juice
- 1 tablespoon cleaved fresh cilantro
- 1 teaspoon unsalted sunflower seeds
- Pinch of crushed red pepper
- ¼ avocado, cut
- Optional side: mixed greens

Directions:

1. In a bowl, mix eggs with milk and salt.
2. Warm 1 teaspoon oil in a nonstick skillet over medium heat. Add the egg blend and cook until the base is set and the inside is still somewhat runny, about 1 to 2 minutes.
3. Flip the omelet over and cook until set, around 30 seconds more.
4. Move to a plate.
5. Mix one tablespoon of oil, kale, lime juice, cilantro, sunflower seeds, crushed red pepper, and a touch of salt.
6. Add kale mix on top of the omelet.
7. As a side, add mixed greens and avocado. Alternately, add the avocado slices to the kale mix.

Easy Egg-White Muffins

Preparation time: 10 minutes

Cooking time: 15 minutes

Servings: 2

Ingredients:

- English muffin
- 2 large egg whites
- Turkey bacon or bacon sausage
- Sharp cheddar cheese or gouda
- Optional ingredients: lettuce, hot sauce, hummus, flax-seeds, or other toppings

Directions:

1. Get a microwavable safe container, then spray to coat with nonstick spray to keep the egg from sticking, then pour egg whites into the dish.
2. Lay turkey bacon or bacon sausage a paper towel for a few minutes and then cook in a skillet.
3. Subsequently, toast your muffin, if preferred.
4. Put the egg dish in the microwave for 30 seconds. Afterward, with a spoon or fork, flip the egg within the dish and cook for another 30 seconds.
5. Whilst the dish remains hot, sprinkle some cheese over the sausage.
6. Use the muffin as a sandwich and add the ingredients inside.
7. You may also add hummus, hot sauce, lettuce, or flax-seeds to your sandwich.

Mushroom Scramble Eggs

Preparation time: 45 minutes

Cooking time: 10 minutes

Servings: 2

Ingredients:

- 2 eggs
- 1 teaspoon turmeric powder
- 1 teaspoon mild curry powder
- 1 ounce kale leaves
- 1 teaspoon extra virgin olive oil
- ½ cup bean stew
- 1 cup mushrooms, equally cut
- Sprinkle of parsley, dry and finely ground
- Optional: Add a seed blend as a topper and some Red Rooster sauce (sriracha sauce) for added flavor.

Directions:

1. Blend the turmeric and curry powder and add some water until a paste is formed.
2. Steam the kale for 2 – 3 minutes.
3. Heat the oil in a skillet over medium heat and fry the bean stew and mushrooms for 2 – 3 minutes until they begin to change color.
4. Add eggs and paste.
5. Cook over a medium heat and then add kale and keep cooking over medium heat for a few minutes.
6. Add the parsley, mix well and serve.

LUNCH RECIPES

Avocado Carbonara

Preparation time: 10 minutes

Cooking time: 10 minutes

Servings: 4

Ingredients:

- 1 large ripe avocado, cut and peeled
- 1 ¾ cups coconut cream
- ½ lemon, juiced
- Salt and black pepper to taste
- 1 tsp freshly minced onion
- 1 tsp freshly minced garlic
- ¼ cup olive oil
- 2 cups spiralized zucchinis
- ⅓ cup grated vegan provolone cheese and some more for garnishing
- 4 tablespoons chopped toasted pine nuts for topping

Directions:

1. In a bowl, mix avocado, coconut cream, lemon juice, minced onion and garlic.
2. Heat olive oil in a large skillet and sauté zucchinis until tender, 5 minutes.
3. Season with a little salt and black pepper.
4. Add avocado mix to the skillet and top it with provolone cheese until the cheese melts and is well coated, for around 5 minutes.
5. Place in a dish, top with more cheese, pine nuts, and serve warm.

Beef Sausage and Spinach Stew

Preparation time: 10 minutes

Cooking time: 25 minutes

Servings: 4

Ingredients:

- 1 pound shredded spinach
- 1 pound beef sausage, crumbled
- 2 garlic cloves, minced
- 1 ½ cups tomatoes, chopped
- 1 cup brown rice, cooked
- 1 cup chopped spring onion
- 1 teaspoon salt
- ¼ teaspoon ground black pepper
- ½ cup fresh cilantro, chopped
- 1 cup meat broth
- 1 tablespoon fennel seeds
- 1 tablespoon cider vinegar

Directions:

1. In a mixing bowl, stir in spinach and fennel seeds. Take half of this mixture to make a layer at the bottom of the pot.
2. In another bowl, mix in rice, sausage, fresh cilantro, spring onion, garlic, salt, and pepper.
3. Add half of this mixture over the spinach mixture and then, top with another layer of the remaining spinach mixture. Finally, top with the remaining part of the meat mixture.
4. In a large-sized mixing bowl, whisk the tomato puree, cider vinegar, and some water. Pour over the mixture.
5. Cover and cook for 30 minutes on medium heat.
6. Serve immediately in individual serving bowls.

No-Fuss Beef Chuck Roast

Preparation time: 10 minutes

Cooking time: 50 minutes

Servings: 6

Ingredients:

- 2 pounds boneless beef chuck roast, trimmed
- ½ pound carrots, peeled and chopped
- 2 pounds Yukon gold potatoes, chopped
- 1 (5 ounce) can beef broth
- 4 minced garlic cloves
- 2 tablespoons olive oil
- ½ pound celery, finely chopped
- 2 bell peppers, sliced
- 1 cup tomato paste
- 2 yellow onions, chopped
- ¼ cup dry white wine
- 1 ½ cups water
- 2 tablespoons all-purpose flour
- ½ teaspoon dried basil
- 1 tablespoon dried thyme
- Kosher salt and ground black pepper for extra flavor

Directions:

1. Using a pressure cooker, heat the oil on sauté mode set to high. Add beef and cook for 3-4 minutes or until it changes color.
2. Pour the beef broth into the cooker.
3. Stir in the onions and garlic, and sauté for another 3 minutes.
4. Stir in the rest of the ingredients except for the flour.
5. Seal the lid and switch the pressure release valve to close. Select pressure cook/manual mode and cook for 50 minutes at high pressure.

6. Once the cooking is complete, do a quick pressure release.
7. Make a slurry by whisking the flour with 1 tbsp. of water.
8. Add to the cooker and place the lid on.
9. Let simmer for about 5 minutes before serving.

Spicy Shredded Beef Roast With Red Wine Sauce

Preparation time: 5 minutes

Cooking time: 45 minutes

Servings: 8

Ingredients:

- 3 pounds beef roast
- ½ cup ketchup
- ½ cup red wine
- 1 cup water
- 2 teaspoons of soy sauce
- 1 tablespoon of brown sugar
- 1 tablespoon of balsamic vinegar
- 2 tablespoons of minced onions
- 1 tablespoon of mustard powder
- 1 teaspoon of chili powder
- 1 teaspoon of minced garlic
- ¼ teaspoon nutmeg
- ½ teaspoon of ground cinnamon
- 1 teaspoon black pepper
- ¼ teaspoon salt
- ¼ teaspoon ginger powder

Directions:

1. Place the beef in your pressure cooker.
2. Whisk together the remaining ingredients in a bowl.
3. Pour this mixture over the beef. Seal the lid and cook for 40 minutes on meat/stew mode at high pressure.
4. When ready, release the pressure gradually, for 10 minutes.

Beef and Tomato Soup

Preparation time: 10 minutes

Cooking time: 10 minutes

Servings: 4

Ingredients:

- 1 cup diced onions
- 1 cup chicken broth
- 1 cup milk
- 1 ½ cups ground beef
- 1 cup of diced tomatoes
- 3 teaspoons of minced garlic
- ¼ cup chopped fresh basil
- 1 tablespoon olive oil

Directions:

1. Heat oil and add the beef. Cook for about 5 minutes or until it changes color.
2. Add onions and garlic, and saute for 2 minutes, until soft.
3. In a blender, blend tomatoes and milk until the mixture becomes smooth.
4. Pour tomato mixture over the beef.
5. Add the rest of the ingredients and stir to combine well.
6. Cover and cook for 30 minutes over medium heat.

The Easiest Sloppy Joes

Preparation time: 10 minutes

Cooking time: 40 minutes

Servings: 8

Ingredients:

- 1 ½ pounds ground beef
- 2 tomatoes, diced
- 8 Kaiser Rolls
- ½ cup barley
- 1 teaspoon chili powder
- 2 tablespoons canola oil
- 2 tablespoons Worcestershire Sauce
- 2 tablespoons tomato ketchup
- 2 tablespoons brown sugar
- 1 cup chopped scallions
- ½ tablespoon cayenne pepper
- 3 cups water

Directions:

1. Add and mix all ingredients in a pressure cooker except for the kaiser rolls.
2. Seal the lid, set it to meat/stew mode and cook for 25 minutes at high pressure.
3. When ready, do a quick pressure release.
4. Divide the mixture between the rolls and serve immediately

Kohlrabi Fries

Preparation time: 10 minutes

Cooking time: 10 minutes

Servings: 6

Ingredients:

- 1 large kohlrabi
- A pinch of pepper salt
- 1 tablespoon paprika powder
- 1 tablespoon olive oil
- 1 teaspoon rosemary

Directions:

1. Preheat the oven to 355°F.
2. Peel the kohlrabi and cut into fries-shaped pieces.
3. Put the oil, paprika, and pepper in a freezer bag. Add the kohlrabi fries and mix everything together well.
4. Cover a baking sheet with parchment paper and then spread the kohlrabi fries on it.
5. Let the fries bake in the oven for half an hour. Sprinkle the fries with salt at the end.

Coconut Thai Curry

Preparation time: 10 minutes

Cooking time: 10 minutes

Servings: 6

Ingredients:

- Chili powder
- Half an eggplant
- 1 carrot
- 1 tablespoon curry powder
- 1 tablespoon curry paste
- Half an onion
- 1 can (200 g) coconut milk
- 1 teaspoon sea salt and pepper
- 9 ounces broccoli
- 1 zucchini
- 1 bell pepper
- ½ cup pineapple
- ½ cup mango
- 2.5 ounces bamboo shoots

Directions:

1. Simmer broccoli for 6 minutes.
2. Cut the fruit into small cubes. Cut the remaining vegetables into equally sized slices.
3. Fry the vegetables and fruits in a little oil for 8 minutes. Season the ingredients as they cook.
4. Add the bamboo shoots and stir in the coconut milk.
5. Simmer for another 10 minutes and at the end season with curry powder, curry, salt and pepper.

Savoy Cabbage Stew

Preparation time: 10 minutes

Cooking time: 10 minutes

Servings: 2

Ingredients:

- 4 ounces savoy cabbage
- 7 ounces carrots
- 7 ounces celery
- ½ teaspoon of coconut oil
- Half a bunch of spring onions
- 2 ounces coconut milk
- Half a red chili pepper
- A stick of lemongrass
- 2 tablespoons lemon juice
- ½ teaspoon vegetable stock
- Pepper and sea salt

Directions:

1. Wash the cabbage and cut into fine pieces with a kitchen knife.
2. Clean carrots and cut into fine sticks. Cut the onions into rings of the same size. Repeat the same with the lemongrass.
3. Cut the red chili in half.
4. Heat the coconut oil in a saucepan.
5. Steam the onions in the pan until soft. After a few minutes, add the honey and mix with the onions. Spices can also be added at this point.
6. Add the kale and simmer for another 2 minutes.
7. Season with salt and pepper. Add the carrots and simmer.
8. Stir in the lemongrass. Then add the water.
9. Let the stew simmer over medium heat for 15

minutes.

10. After 5 minutes, add the coconut milk and the chili halves to the saucepan.
11. Season with lemon juice before serving.

Beautiful Tomato Meatballs

Preparation time: 30 minutes

Servings: 4

Ingredients:

For meatballs:

- 1 pound ground beef
- ½ cup breadcrumbs
- ½ diced onion
- 1 teaspoon of minced garlic
- 1 egg
- 1 teaspoon dried parsley
- 1 teaspoon dried thyme
- ½ teaspoon salt and black pepper for added flavor
- 1 ½ cups tomato juice

Other ingredients:

- 1 cup canned peeled diced tomatoes
- 1 tablespoon brown sugar
- ¼ teaspoon garlic powder
- ¼ teaspoon dried oregano
- Cooking spray to grease

Directions:

1. Combine the first 9 ingredients for the meatballs in a bowl. Mix well.
2. Shape the mixture into meatballs.
3. Coat the pressure cooker with cooking spray.
4. Place meatballs in the cooker and brown them for a few minutes, on sauté mode at high pressure.
5. Stir in the remaining ingredients.
6. Seal the lid and cook for 20 minutes on meat/stew at high pressure.
7. When ready, release the pressure quickly and serve

hot.

Chickpea Stew With Red Onion and Tomatoes

Preparation time: 10 minutes

Cooking time: 35 minutes

Servings: 4

Ingredients:

- 6 oz chickpeas, soaked overnight
- 2 tomatoes, peeled and chopped
- 1 red onion, chopped
- 1 tablespoon cumin seeds
- 2 cups vegetable broth
- 2 tablespoon olive oil
- 2 tablespoon melted butter
- 2 tablespoon freshly chopped parsley
- ½ teaspoon salt and black pepper for added flavor

Directions:

1. In a pressure cooker, add in the olive oil, tomatoes, onion, cumin seeds, chickpeas, and pour in the broth. Seal the lid and set the steam handle.
2. Cook broth for 30 minutes on high pressure. Do a quick release and set aside to cool for a while.
3. Transfer the stew to a food processor and season with salt and pepper.
4. Process until pureed and ladle to a serving dish.
5. Stir in 2 tablespoons of butter. Garnish with freshly chopped parsley.

Spanish-Style "Tortilla de Patatas"

Preparation time: 10 minutes

Cooking time: 20 minutes

Servings: 3

Ingredients:

- 5 eggs, beaten
- 1 cup spinach, torn, rinsed
- 1 potato, chopped
- 1 cup heavy cream
- Salt and black pepper to taste
- ¼ teaspoon dried thyme
- 1 tablespoon olive oil

Directions:

1. In a bowl, mix eggs, heavy cream, and potato.
2. Sprinkle with salt and black pepper, and stir to combine.
3. Heat oil to sauté and cook the spinach and thyme for 3 minutes, or until wilted. Remove the spinach from the pot.
4. Stir the spinach into the previously prepared mixture.
5. Transfer all to an oven-safe dish that fits in the instant pot.
6. Insert the trivet and pour 1 cup of water, then place the oven-safe dish on top.
7. Seal the lid and cook on high pressure for 20 minutes.
8. Release the steam naturally, for 5 minutes.

Pork Casserole

Preparation time: 10 minutes

Cooking time: 45 minutes

Servings: 4

Ingredients:

- 1 pound pork, ground
- 2 shallots, chopped
- 2 garlic cloves, minced
- 1 tablespoon olive oil
- 2 red bell peppers, roughly cubed
- 2 tomatoes, cubed
- 1 cup mozzarella, shredded
- 2 tablespoons parsley, chopped
- Salt and black pepper to the taste

Directions:

1. Preheat the oven to 380°F.
2. Add oil to a pan on medium heat. Add the shallots and the garlic and sauté for 5 minutes.
3. Add the meat, bell peppers and the tomatoes, stir and cook for 5 minutes more.
4. Spread this into a casserole dish, sprinkle the mozzarella and the parsley on top, place in the oven and cook at 380°F for 35 minutes.
5. Divide the mix between plates and serve.

Leeks and Eggs Mix

Preparation time: 5 minutes

Cooking time: 15 minutes

Servings: 4

Ingredients:

- 3 leeks, sliced
- 8 eggs, whisked
- 1 tablespoon avocado oil
- ¼ cup almond milk
- ¼ teaspoon garlic powder
- 1 teaspoon sweet paprika
- 1 tablespoon cilantro, chopped
- Salt and black pepper to the taste

Directions:

1. Heat up a pan with the oil over medium heat, add the leeks, garlic powder, and the paprika, stir and sauté for 5 minutes.
2. Add the eggs mixed with the milk, salt and pepper. Stir and cook for 10 minutes more.
3. Divide between plates, sprinkle the cilantro on top and serve.

Broccoli and Eggs Salad

Preparation time: 10 minutes

Cooking time: 0 minutes

Servings: 4

Ingredients:

- 1 pound broccoli florets, steamed
- 4 eggs, hard boiled, peeled and cut into wedges
- 2 spring onions, chopped
- ½ teaspoon chili powder
- 1 tablespoon olive oil
- 1 tablespoon lime juice
- Salt and black pepper to the taste

Directions:

1. In a bowl, combine the broccoli with the eggs and the other ingredients.
2. Serve immediately or pre-chilled.

DINNER RECIPES

Salmon Stew

Preparation Time: 8 minutes

Cooking Time: 12 minutes

Servings: 2

Ingredients:

- 1-pound salmon fillet, sliced
- 1 onion, chopped
- A pinch of salt
- 1 tablespoon butter, melted
- 1 cup fish broth
- ½ teaspoon red chili powder

Directions:

1. Season the salmon fillets with salt and red chili powder.
2. Put butter and onions in a skillet and sauté for about 3 minutes.
3. Add seasoned salmon and cook for about 2 minutes on each side.
4. Add fish broth and secure the lid.
5. Cook for about 7 minutes on medium heat and open the lid.
6. Dish out and serve immediately.
7. Alternately, transfer the stew in a bowl and set aside to cool for meal prepping. Divide the mixture into 2 containers. Cover the containers and refrigerate for up to 2 days. Reheat in the microwave before serving.

Sweet and Sour Fish

Preparation Time: 15 minutes

Cooking Time: 10 minutes

Servings: 2

Ingredients:

- ¼ cup butter, melted
- 1 pound fish chunks
- 2 drops stevia
- 1 tablespoon vinegar
- Salt and black pepper for extra flavor

Directions:

1. Pour the butter in a skillet, add the fish chunks and cook for about 3 minutes.
2. Add stevia, vinegar, salt, and black pepper. Continue cooking for about 10 minutes while stirring continuously.
3. Plate into bowls and serve immediately.
4. Alternately, place the fish in a container and let cool for meal prepping. Separate it into 2 containers and refrigerate for up to 2 days.
5. Reheat in the microwave before serving.

Paprika Butter Shrimp

Preparation Time: 15 minutes

Cooking Time: 15 minutes

Servings: 2

Ingredients:

- ¼ tablespoon smoked paprika
- 1 tablespoon sour cream
- ½ pound shrimps
- 1/8 cup butter
- Salt and black pepper for extra flavor

Directions:

1. Preheat the oven to 390°F and grease a baking dish.
2. Mix together all the ingredients in a large bowl and transfer into the baking dish.
3. Place in the oven and bake for about 15 minutes.
4. Place the paprika-seasoned shrimp in a dish and let cool for meal prepping.
5. Separate it into 2 containers and cover with the lids. Refrigerate for 1-2 days and reheat in the microwave before serving.

Almond Flour Burger With Goat Cheese

Preparation Time: 10 minutes

Cooking Time: 20 minutes

Servings: 2

Ingredients:

- 2 almond flour bagels
- 2 tablespoons of fresh goat cheese
- 4 slices smoked salmon
- 1 teaspoon salt and pepper
- 4 radishes
- Dill

Directions:

1. Cut the gluten-free bagels in half. Put the two halves in the toaster to make them crisp.
2. Spread both slices with fresh goat cheese and add salmon.
3. Garnish the bagel with the radish and dill.
4. A pinch of salt and pepper and it's ready
5. If meal prepping, put each burger in a container and store in the refrigerator

Sausage Skillet With Cabbage

Preparation Time: 5 minutes

Cooking Time: 13 minutes

Servings: 2

Ingredients:

- 1 tablespoon olive oil
- ¾ cup shredded green cabbage
- ¾ cup grated red cabbage
- ¼ cup diced onion
- ¼ cup spicy sausages
- ¼ cup grated mozzarella
- 1 tablespoon fresh and chopped parsley
- A pinch of salt and pepper to taste

Directions:

1. Place a large skillet on a stove over medium-high heat and heat olive oil. Coat the cabbage and onion in the heated oil. Let heat for about 8-10 minutes or until vegetables are tender.
2. Chop the sausage into bite-size pieces. Mix with cabbage and onion and let heat for another 8 minutes.
3. Spread the cheese over the top
4. Cover the skillet with a lid and set aside for 5 minutes to melt.
5. Remove the lid and mix your ingredients together. Garnish with salt, pepper, and parsley before serving.
6. To assemble the dish, divide the mixture between 2 containers. Store it in the refrigerator for up to 2 days if you are meal prepping.

Chicken and Broccoli Gratin

Preparation Time: 10 minutes

Cooking Time: 10 minutes

Servings: 4

Ingredients:

- 1 pound of chicken breasts
- ¼ cup almond butter
- 32 ounces of fresh cream
- 1 cup goat cheese
- 2 organic eggs
- 2 crushed garlic cloves
- A pinch of salt
- A pinch of pepper

Directions:

1. Preheat the oven to 390°F.
2. Cook the broccoli in a pot of water for 10 minutes. It must remain firm.
3. Melt the butter in a skillet; add the crushed garlic clove and the salted and peppered chicken. Sauté until it turns a brown color.
4. Drain the broccoli and mix with the chicken.
5. Beat the eggs with the cream, salt, and pepper. Place broccoli and chicken in a baking dish, cover with cream mixture and sprinkle with grated cheese.
6. Put in the oven at 390°F for 20 minutes.
7. When the gratin is ready, set it aside to cool for 3 minutes.
8. Cut the gratin into two halves or in four portions.
9. Place each two portions of gratin in separate containers.

Chicken Curry

Preparation Time: 10 minutes

Cooking Time: 30 minutes

Servings: 2

Ingredients:

- 2 chicken breasts
- 1 garlic clove
- 1 small onion
- 1 zucchini
- 2 carrots
- 1 box of bamboo shoots or sprouts
- 1 cup coconut milk
- 1 tablespoon tomato paste
- 2 tablespoons yellow curry paste

Directions:

1. Mince the onion and sauté in a pan with a little oil for a few minutes.
2. Add chicken cut in large cubes and crushed garlic, salt, pepper and sauté quickly over high heat until the meat begins to turn white.
3. Pour zucchini and carrots in thick slices into the pan.
4. Sear over high heat for a few minutes, then add the coconut milk, tomato sauce, bamboo shoots and one to two tablespoons curry paste, depending on your taste.
5. Cook over low heat and cover for 30 to 45 minutes, stirring occasionally
6. Once cooked, divide the chicken curry between 2 containers.
7. Store the containers in the refrigerator.

Spinach Chicken

Preparation Time: 10 minutes

Cooking Time: 10 minutes

Servings: 2

Ingredients:

- 2 garlic cloves, minced
- 2 tablespoons unsalted butter, divided
- ¼ cup parmesan cheese, shredded
- ¾ pound chicken tenders
- ¼ cup heavy cream
- 10 ounces frozen spinach, chopped
- Salt and black pepper, to taste

Directions:

1. Heat one tablespoon of butter in a large skillet and add chicken, salt, and black pepper.
2. Cook for about 3 minutes on both sides and transfer the chicken to a bowl.
3. Melt remaining butter in the skillet and add garlic, cheese, heavy cream, and spinach.
4. Cook for about 2 minutes and add the chicken.
5. Cook for about 5 minutes on low heat and dish out to immediately serve.
6. Alternately, place the chicken in a bowl and let cool for meal prepping. Separate it into 2 containers and close the lids.
7. Refrigerate for up to 3 days and reheat in the microwave before serving.

Lemongrass Prawns

Preparation Time: 10 minutes + 2 hours marinating

Cooking Time: 15 minutes

Servings: 2

Ingredients:

- ½ red chili pepper, seeded and chopped
- 2 lemongrass stalks
- ½ pound prawns, deveined and peeled
- 6 tablespoons butter
- ¼ teaspoon smoked paprika

Directions:

1. Preheat the oven to 390°F and grease a baking dish.
2. Mix together red chili pepper, butter, smoked paprika and prawns in a bowl.
3. Marinate for about 2 hours and then thread the prawns on the lemongrass stalks.
4. Arrange the threaded prawns on the baking dish and place in the oven.
5. Bake for about 15 minutes and dish out to serve immediately.
6. Alternately, place the prawns in a dish and let cool for meal prepping.
7. Separate it into 2 containers and close the lids. Refrigerate for up to 4 days and reheat in the microwave before serving.

Stuffed Mushrooms

Preparation Time: 20 minutes

Cooking Time: 25 minutes

Servings: 4

Ingredients:

- 2 ounces bacon, crumbled
- ½ tablespoon butter
- ¼ teaspoon paprika powder
- 2 portobello mushrooms
- 1 ounce cream cheese
- ¾ tablespoon fresh chives, chopped
- A pinch of salt and black pepper for extra flavor

Directions:

1. Preheat the oven to 400°F and grease a baking dish.
2. Heat butter in a skillet and add mushrooms.
3. Sauté for about 4 minutes and set aside.
4. Mix together cream cheese, chives, paprika powder, salt, and black pepper in a bowl.
5. Stuff the mushrooms with this mixture and transfer on the baking dish.
6. Place in the oven and bake for about 20 minutes.
7. These mushrooms can be refrigerated for about 3 days for meal prepping and can be served with scrambled eggs.

Jamaican Curry Chicken Drumsticks

Preparation Time: 5 minutes

Cooking Time: 20 minutes

Servings: 4

Ingredients:

- 1 ½ pounds chicken drumsticks
- 1 tablespoon Jamaican curry powder
- 1 teaspoon salt
- 1 cup chicken broth
- ½ medium onion, diced
- ½ teaspoon dried thyme

Directions:

1. Sprinkle the salt and curry powder over the chicken drumsticks.
2. Place the chicken drumsticks into the Instant Pot, along with the remaining ingredients.
3. Secure the lid. Select the Manual mode and set the cooking time for 20 minutes at High Pressure.
4. Once cooking is complete, do a quick pressure release. Carefully open the lid. Serve warm.

Chicken Fillets With Cheese Sauce

Preparation Time: 5 minutes

Cooking Time: 10 minutes

Servings: 4

Ingredients:

- 1 tablespoon olive oil
- 1 pound chicken fillets
- ½ teaspoon dried basil
- 1 cup chicken broth

Cheese Sauce:

- 3 teaspoons butter, at room temperature
- ⅓ cup grated Gruyère cheese
- ⅓ cup Neufchâtel cheese, at room temperature
- ⅓ cup heavy cream
- 3 tablespoons unsweetened coconut milk
- 1 teaspoon shallot powder
- ½ teaspoon granulated garlic
- ½ teaspoon of salt and black pepper for extra flavor

Directions:

1. Set your Instant Pot to Sauté and heat the olive oil until sizzling.
2. Add the chicken and sear each side for 3 minutes. Sprinkle it with basil, salt, and black pepper.
3. Pour the broth into the Instant Pot and stir well.
4. Lock the lid. Select the Manual mode and set the cooking time for 6 minutes at High Pressure.
5. When the timer beeps, perform a natural pressure release for 10 minutes, then release any remaining pressure. Carefully remove the lid.
6. Transfer the chicken to a platter and set aside.
7. Clean the Instant Pot. Press the Sauté button and melt the butter.
8. Add the cheeses, heavy cream, milk, shallot powder,

and garlic, stirring until everything is heated through.
9. Pour the cheese sauce over the chicken and serve.

SNACK RECIPES

Vanilla Berry Meringues

Preparation Time: 15 minutes

Cooking Time: 2 hours 0 minutes

Servings: 10

Ingredients:

- 1 teaspoon vanilla extract
- 3 tablespoons freeze-dried mixed berries, crushed
- 3 large egg whites, at room temperature
- ⅓ cup erythritol
- 1 teaspoon lemon rind

Directions:

1. In a mixing bowl, beat the egg whites until foamy.
2. Add in vanilla extract, lemon rind, and erythritol; continue to mix, using an electric mixer, until stiff and glossy.
3. Add the crushed berries and mix again until well combined. Use two teaspoons to spoon meringue onto parchment-lined cookie sheets.
4. Bake at 220°F for about 1 hour 45 minutes. The meringue should lift easily off the baking sheet when done. If it does not, continue baking while checking every few minutes.

Chocolate Cake

Preparation Time: 15 minutes

Cooking Time: 40 minutes

Servings: 10

Ingredients:

- 5 eggs
- ½ teaspoon ground cinnamon
- ½ cup water
- ¾ cup erythritol
- 14 ounces chocolate
- 2 sticks butter, unsweetened and cold
- A pinch of coarse salt

For Peanut-Choc Ganache:

- 9 ounces chocolate, unsweetened
- ¼ cup smooth peanut butter
- ¾ cups whipped cream
- A pinch of coarse salt

Directions

1. In a medium-sized pan, bring the water to a boil; add in the erythritol and let it simmer until it has dissolved.
2. Melt the chocolate and butter; beat the mixture with an electric mixer. Add the chocolate mixture to the hot water mixture.
3. Fold in the eggs, one at a time, beating continuously.
4. Add in the cinnamon and salt, and stir well to combine.
5. Spoon the mixture into a parchment-lined baking pan and wrap with foil.
6. Lower the baking pan into a larger pan that is filled with hot water about 1 inch deep. Bake in the pre-

heated oven at 365°F for about 45 minutes. Meanwhile, place the whipped cream in a pan over a moderately-high heat and bring to a boil.

7. Pour the hot cream over the chocolate and whisk to combine. Add in the peanut butter and salt; continue to mix until creamy and smooth.

8. Glaze your cake and place in the refrigerator until set.

American-Style Mini Cheesecakes

Preparation Time: 15 minutes

Cooking Time: 25 minutes

Servings: 12

Ingredients:

- 6 ounces Neufchatel cheese, at room temperature
- 7 tablespoons coconut oil, melted
- 5 eggs
- ¼ teaspoon ground cinnamon
- ¼ cup Swerve
- 2 ounces cocoa powder, unsweetened
- 1 teaspoon vanilla paste
- 1 teaspoon rum extract
- ⅓ teaspoon baking powder

Directions:

1. Preheat the oven to 350°F.
2. Beat the ingredients using your electric mixer on high speed.
3. Line a mini muffin pan with 12 liners.
4. Spoon the mixture into prepared muffins cups.
5. Bake in the preheated oven at 350°F for about 20 minutes. Bon appétit.

Classic Chocolate Bars

Preparation Time: 5 minutes

Cooking Time: 25 minutes

Servings: 10

Ingredients:

- ½ stick butter, cold
- 1 ½ cups whipped cream
- 8 ounces chocolate chunks, sugar-free
- ¼ teaspoon cinnamon
- ½ teaspoon rum extract
- 1 teaspoon vanilla extract
- ¼ cup coconut flour
- ¼ cup flaxseed meal
- 1 cup almond meal
- 2 packets stevia
- A pinch of coarse salt

Directions:

1. Start by preheating your oven to 340°F.
2. Coat a baking dish with a piece of parchment paper.
3. Add the coconut flour, flaxseed meal, almond meal, stevia, cinnamon, rum extract, vanilla, and salt to your blender.
4. Blend until everything is well incorporated.
5. Cut in the cold butter and continue to blend until well combined.
6. Spoon the batter into the bottom of the prepared baking pan.
7. Bake for 12 to 15 minutes and place on a wire rack to cool slightly.
8. Bring the whipped cream to a simmer; add in the chocolate chunks and whisk to combine. Spread the chocolate filling over the crust and place in your refriger-

ator until set. Cut into bars.

Hard-Boiled Eggs Stuffed With Ricotta Cheese

Preparation Time: 15 minutes

Cooking Time: 30 minutes

Servings: 8

Ingredients:

- 4 eggs
- 1 tablespoon green tabasco
- 2 tablespoon Greek yogurt
- 2 tablespoon ricotta cheese
- Salt to taste

Directions:

1. Cover the eggs with salted water and bring to a boil over medium heat for 10 minutes.
2. Place the eggs in an ice bath and let cool for 10 minutes. Peel and slice in half lengthwise.
3. Scoop out the yolks to a bowl; mash with a fork.
4. Whisk together the tabasco, Greek yogurt, ricotta cheese, mashed yolks, and salt, in a bowl.
5. Spoon this mixture into the egg white.
6. Arrange on a serving plate to serve.

Chocolate Ganache

Preparation Time: 6 minutes

Cooking Time: 10 minutes

Servings: 4

Ingredients:

- ½ cup heavy cream
- 4 ounces dark chocolate, unsweetened, and chopped

Directions

1. Put the cream into a pan and heat up over medium heat.
2. Take off the heat when it begins to simmer, add the chocolate pieces, and stir until it melts.
3. Serve cold.

No Bake Chocolate Peanut Butter Bars

Preparation Time: 10 minutes

Cooking Time: 40 minutes

Servings: 4

Ingredients:

- 2 cups peanut butter, divided into 1 ¼ cups and ¾ cups
- ¾ cup butter, softened
- 2 cups powdered sugar
- 3 cups graham cracker crumbs
- 1 (12 ounce) package Semi-Sweet Chocolate Mini Morsels, divided

Directions:

1. Grease 9x13 inch baking pan.
2. In a big mixer bowl, whip butter and 1 ¼ cups of peanut butter till it becomes creamy. Slowly whip in one cup of powdered sugar.
3. Work in the half cup morsels, graham cracker crumbs and leftover powdered sugar using a wooden spoon or your hands.
4. Press evenly into the prepared baking pan. Use a spatula to smooth out the top.
5. In a medium-sized and heavy-duty saucepan on the lowest possible heat, melt leftover morsels and leftover peanut butter while mixing continuously till smooth in consistency.
6. Spread on top of graham cracker crust in the pan. Let chill in the refrigerator till chocolate becomes firm, for no less than 60 minutes; chop into bars. Keep in the fridge.

Butter Fat Bombs

Preparation Time: 5 minutes

Cooking Time: 12 minutes

Servings: 12

Ingredients:

- 2 cups heavy whipping cream (cold)
- 1 teaspoon vanilla
- 2 to 3 tablespoons sweetener to taste
- 3 tablespoons peanut butter

Directions:

1. Put the chilled whipping cream in a medium mixing bowl and mix at medium speed.
2. Add the vanilla to that. Once a soft peak has been reached, add the sugar replacement followed by the peanut butter.
3. Whip till it is thoroughly mixed.
4. Insert 12 cupcake liners in a muffin pan.
5. Use a plastic bag or icing tube to squeeze the peanut butter mix into the liners.
6. Place in the freezer for 2 hours or until frozen. Then place in a sealed container in the freezer for storage.

Chocolate Fat Bombs

Preparation Time: 8 minutes

Cooking Time: 12 minutes

Servings: 2

Ingredients:

- ½ cup coconut oil
- ½ cup brown sugar
- ½ cup peanut butter
- ¾ cup chocolate chips
- Sea salt, if desired

Directions:

1. Heat a medium saucepan over medium-low heat.
2. Add the coconut oil and wait until it has fully melted.
3. Add the sugar replacement, the peanut butter, and the chocolate chips.
4. Stir the mixture constantly until it has melted fully.
5. Remove from heat and allow the mixture to cool for 5-10 minutes.
6. Carefully spoon into a silicone mini muffin jar until each muffin is ¾ full.
7. Sprinkle with sea salt (optional)
8. Freeze until firm.

Smores

Preparation Time: 5 minutes

Cooking Time: 15 minutes

Servings: 6

Ingredients:

- 12 Graham Crackers
- 6 squares Lindt 90% Dark Chocolate
- 6 keto marshmallows

Directions:

1. Put six crackers on a cookie sheet lined with parchment paper, cover each with a chocolate square.
2. Bake or broil for 3-5 minutes until the chocolate has melted.
3. Cover each one with a marshmallow, accompanied by another graham cracker. Enjoy immediately.

Spicy Tuna Mousse

Preparation time: 15 minutes

Cooking time: 25 minutes

Servings: 5

Ingredients:

- 1 ½ teaspoons powdered gelatin
- 3 tablespoons water
- 2 ounces mascarpone cheese
- ⅓ teaspoon grated fresh ginger
- ¼ teaspoon freshly ground black pepper
- ½ teaspoon celery salt
- 1 teaspoon minced jalapeno
- 1 minced garlic clove
- ¼ cup finely chopped shallots
- 3 ounces flaked canned tuna
- 3 tablespoons mayonnaise
- 1 teaspoon Dijon mustard

Directions:

1. Put the gelatin in the water and let it dissolve. Let it stand for 10 minutes.
2. In a pan over medium heat, melt the mascarpone. Stir in the gelatin and whisk together.
3. Cool the mixture and then add the ginger, black pepper, celery salt, jalapeno, garlic, shallots, tuna, mayonnaise and mustard.
4. Put the mixture in 5 mousse molds and refrigerate overnight.
5. When ready to serve, invert the molds over individual plates.

Jazzed-Up Olives

Preparation Time: 5 minutes

Cooking Time: 4 minutes

Servings: 8

Ingredients:

- ½ cup extra-virgin olive oil
- 2 garlic cloves, minced
- 2 teaspoons fresh thyme leaves
- 1 teaspoon dried oregano
- ½ teaspoon red pepper flakes
- 2 cups mixed olives
- 1 tablespoon freshly squeezed lemon juice

Directions:

1. In a skillet, warm the olive oil over low heat. Add the garlic, thyme, oregano, and red pepper flakes and cook for about 2 minutes until the garlic starts to turn golden.
2. Add the olives and stir for about 1 minute to coat them in the oil mixture.
3. Transfer the olive mixture, including the oil, to a bowl and toss with the lemon juice. Allow to marinate at room temperature for 1 hour before serving.

Hummus Dip

Preparation Time: 5 minutes

Cooking Time: 10 minutes

Servings: 4

Ingredients:

- 1 cup classic hummus
- ½ cup finely chopped tomatoes ¼ cup shredded Fontina cheese
- 2 tablespoons chopped pitted kalamata olives
- 1 tablespoon Sweet Hot Cherry Pepper Relish

Directions:

1. Spread the hummus in the bottom of a small serving bowl.
2. Cover the hummus with the chopped tomatoes. Add a layer of cheese, followed by a layer of kalamata olives.
3. Spoon the cherry pepper relish in the center to add as desired.

Spicy Chickpeas

Preparation Time: 5 minutes

Cooking Time: 10 minutes

Servings: 6

Ingredients:

- 1 (15-ounce) can chickpeas, rinsed and drained
- 2 tablespoons extra-virgin olive oil
- 1 teaspoon paprika
- ½ teaspoon salt
- ½ teaspoon cayenne pepper

Directions:

1. Pat the chickpeas dry with a paper towel. Remove as many of the soft skins as you can.
2. In a large skillet, heat the olive oil over low heat. Add the chickpeas and stir to coat. Slowly toast the chickpeas, occasionally stirring, until they get a little crunchy, about 10 minutes.
3. Using a slotted spoon, transfer the chickpeas to a bowl lined with paper towels to absorb any excess oil.
4. Transfer the chickpeas to a serving bowl, sprinkle with the paprika, salt, and cayenne, and toss to coat.

Croquettes

Preparation Time: 1 hour 30 minutes

Cooking Time: 40 minutes

Servings: 12

Ingredients:

For the kibbeh dough:

- 1 ½ cups fine bulgur
- 2 cups warm water
- 1 ½ pounds ground beef
- 1 onion, cut into chunks
- 2 teaspoons ground allspice
- 1 teaspoon ground coriander
- 1 teaspoon freshly ground black pepper
- ½ teaspoon ground cinnamon
- Pinch of salt

For the stuffing:

- 2 tablespoons extra-virgin olive oil
- 1 onion, finely chopped
- 8 ounces ground beef or lamb
- ½ teaspoon ground allspice
- ¼ teaspoon ground cinnamon
- Pinch freshly ground black pepper
- Pinch of salt

Directions:

To make the dough:

1. In a bowl, combine the bulgur and warm water and soak for 15 minutes. Drain. Wrap the bulgur in a kitchen towel and squeeze out the excess water.
2. In a food processor, combine the ground beef, onion, allspice, coriander, pepper, cinnamon, and salt. Process until the mixture forms a paste.
3. Transfer the mixture to a bowl and add the bulgur. Mix

by hand to form a dough. Cover and refrigerate while you make the stuffing.

To make the stuffing:

1. Place a large skillet over medium heat and add the olive oil. Next, add the onion and sauté for about 3 minutes, until it starts to soften.
2. Add the ground meat and cook for 5 to 7 minutes, until cooked through.
3. Add the allspice, cinnamon, salt, and pepper and stir to combine. Take off the heat and let cool.
4. Set up an assembly line with a bowl of water, the bowl of kibbeh dough, and the bowl of stuffing. Line a rimmed baking sheet with parchment paper.
5. Dampen your hands with water. Shape 2 tablespoons of dough into a flat disc. Wrap 1 tablespoon of stuffing inside the dough. Pinch to close.
6. Continue until you use all the ingredients, wetting your hands before forming each one. Place the kibbeh on the prepared baking sheet and refrigerate for 1 hour. Preheat the oven to 350°F.
7. Bake for 30 to 35 minutes, until golden brown.

CONCLUSION

"I don't have time" is a wonderful phrase.

Suddenly, you have the perfect excuse for everything you do not get around to doing, and for everything you did not achieve: "I'd love to, but I don't have time." Be honest with yourself: Is this a reason or an excuse?

When you say, "I don't have time," you are giving yourself permission not to do things. Whether it is exercising, losing weight, or cooking a healthy dinner, it is often an excuse and not the real reason.

It looks very different if you say, "It's not a high-enough priority." This immediately puts it right back as your own responsibility, and you have to ask yourself honestly, "Do I really want this enough to find the time for it?" You need to prioritize your tasks on a daily basis. If you want something enough, the time will be there, and your planning will encompass it; do not forget, planning is a habit. Keep in mind, any action that is repeatedly done over a period of 40 days will turn into a habit.

When planning becomes part of your everyday routine, you will notice that many things you usually do can be reduced to take less time, which will free up extra time to be able to do things that you could not do before.

You can find time if you want to. It is simply a matter of priorities. Every minute of the day, all of us are putting our main priorities first. It is important that you decide what your priorities are and how you are benefiting from them.

The reality is that we often end up wasting time by not knowing what it is we want to achieve. Because of this, we fill in a lot of our time with whatever's at hand, such as checking our social media, and cannot fit in what we would really prefer to be doing. By being more mindful of your goals and the things you want to achieve in your life, no matter how big or how small, you will be able to find the time to take small steps towards achieving them. Any progress is good, whether it is small or large, fast or slow.

The best way to keep yourself on track is to make an activity list at the start of the week. Planning ahead is crucial. This should include both the things you need to do and the things you want to do, assigning an appropriate amount of time for each activity. You can use any format that is convenient, but handwriting a list helps it stick in your memory and also gives you a good point of reference to look back on when you need a boost of motivation. It is normal to have lapses in motivation as you go through a working week, after all.

Of course, your week is not always going to go according to plan, but if you have a schedule, it is a lot easier to readjust without forgetting what you really want to do. Planning helps you to focus and gives structure to the path ahead. Knowing the path you need to take will help you put your priorities in order of importance. This is hugely important when you feel overwhelmed with responsibilities and a lot is going on in your life. This will help you feel less stressed and also help you find some free time within your busy schedule.

Often, it is the stress of feeling short of time that makes that very lack of time worse, since it drains your energy. That means taking time out to feel good can give you back more time, and therefore increase your productivity levels in whatever you are focusing on.

This could be improving your health with exercise or healthy eating. It could be improving your mental state with yoga or meditation. It could be energizing yourself with a hobby you love, or spending time with friends or family that stimulate you. It could simply be getting enough sleep. Whatever you need to do to feel good could help you find the extra time you need for your other activities.

We are all procrastinators at times. We delay completing certain tasks, and we put things off; instead of doing something today, we leave it for tomorrow. But why do we do it? How do we benefit from this behavior? There must be a reason for behaving this way, surely?

Edward Young, an English poet living in the 18th century, said that procrastination is the thief of time. I agree with this statement. We start doing something, but do not finish it. We leave it for the next day or the next week. Before you know it, a huge amount of time has passed and that task, the one which began as routine, is now hugely urgent. That causes stress and panic, two things that are extremely detrimental to your health and well-being.

We procrastinate for different reasons. Sometimes we procrastinate because we want to be perfect and want to do everything right, but we believe that we cannot do it the way we ought to do it. Sometimes we procrastinate to put off tasks that are not pleasurable. At other times we are too scared of failure, and sometimes we are even scared of success, so we avoid doing things that we are supposed to be doing.

Whatever the reason is, we try to hide from our emotions by delaying the process, so that we do not need to feel a certain way. You could say that procrastination is there to keep us safe, to protect us from certain emotions, but on the other hand, procrastination can steal our joy and peace, bring anxiety, and make us worried. Feeling this way can make us feel drained and negative about life. It is far better to avoid procrastination as much as possible, to kick its negative effects out of your life.

Procrastination can cause lots of stress. This is especially bad if you have too much happening on an everyday basis. Procrastination is bad for your mental health and can affect your self-esteem and self-confidence, as well as introducing the feeling of guilt. Seeing everyone else progressing when you feel stuck and unable to move forward is not a nice feeling to have, and it is one that is likely to sap away your confidence and make you wonder why nothing you try ever goes the way you plan.

Put simply, when you procrastinate, you are leaving things to be done later. You are leaving things for another time, another day, another month. This will just add more frustration and stress to your already busy life, as you will not be achieving things that you want to achieve or completing tasks that you need to complete. This will not help you feel less busy; it will actually add more business to your already busy life.

Be honest with yourself. Ask yourself how motivated you are to achieve the goals you are working towards. Without motivation, your energy will be low, and you will postpone jobs, both big and small, for another time. Procrastination will make you feel even busier in the end, not to mention far more stressed.

Here are some of the ways to deal with procrastination:

- Prioritize the most important things, and do them first thing in the morning. Piling up jobs to do later will cause more stress.
- Recognize what procrastination is trying to protect you from.
- Plan in advance so that you can make the time for things that need doing.
- Set time limits for your tasks, but do not be too hard on yourself if you go over by a couple of minutes.

We all want to be healthy; who would not want that? The problem is that many people believe that their busy lifestyle does not allow them to find time to look after their health. But healthy living does not have to mean spending hours in the gym or preparing insanely complex meals. All it takes is to make it important enough to you, and soon you will find that you have all the time you need for a healthy lifestyle.

Exercising when you do not have time is hard for many people, but exercise is not separate from the rest of your life, and you do not necessarily have to set aside a long stretch of time to do it. If you can manage an hour in the gym every day, that is fine; otherwise, you can simply spend a few minutes doing simple stretches each time you stop for a break.

Similarly, healthy walking or cycling can be built into your daily routine. Even if you have a long daily commute, arranging it to include a five-minute walk should not be too difficult. Could you perhaps walk down to the local shops in less than the time it would take you to drive to the supermarket?

Something that I often suggest my clients do is to stand up or walk while you are talking on the phone. I have noticed that people often sit down in order to speak on the phone, but actually, if you spend that time walking around, it helps the number of steps you do daily add up. Remember: one step at a time.

Being busy or lacking time should never be a reason for eating unhealthy, certainly when it comes to snacks. Many healthy snacks, such as fruit, nuts, or vegetable sticks, for instance, take no longer to prepare than grabbing a chocolate bar or a bag of crisps. You just need to be organized so that you have healthy snacks on hand when you need them.

One of the ways to deal with this is to always carry healthy snacks with you, such as have a bag of nuts or seeds in your handbag, or have a banana in your gym bag, or have a healthy protein bar in your car, or have a bag of oatmeal cakes in your desk at the office. Knowing that you have something healthy on hand will stop you from buying a chocolate bar or ice cream while paying for the gasoline or catching a morning train to work.

Many people complain about lack of time when it comes to preparing meals. My experience is that preparing a healthy meal does not need to take longer than ordering a pizza or heating up a ready meal from the supermarket. Keep a folder of healthy and quick recipes to call on when you need them or simply go on the internet and type "quick and healthy recipes" — you will find lots of them there. Alternatively, you can have your own healthy ready meals available by preparing and freezing them when you do have time. Of course, drinking plenty of water takes no extra time at all.

Getting enough good quality sleep is a must. Ensuring that you have around eight hours sleep each night is likely to give you that time back. You will be more energized during the day and get through your schedule more quickly. Similarly, periodically taking five or ten minutes to meditate will improve your performance.

Healthy living is about the mind and emotions too, and it is important to have a social life that will boost your mental state. You do not need extra time for this; however, simply save your social time for people and activities that will help, not hinder, your aim of healthy living.

REFERENCES

5 Bad Eating Habits and How to Break Them. (2018, December 12). Eating-Well. https://www.eatingwell.com/article/77961/5-bad-eating-habits-and-how-to-break-them

Bouchez, C. (n.d.). How to Drop Pound-Packing Habits. WebMD. Retrieved February 11, 2021, from https://www.webmd.com/diet/obesity/features/how-to-drop-pound-packing-habits

Easy Healthy Recipes - Best Healthy Meal Ideas - Delish.com. (n.d.). Delish. Retrieved February 11, 2021, from https://www.delish.com/healthy-recipes

Food Network UK | TV Channel | Easy Recipes, TV Shows. (2020). Search Page. Food Network UK | TV Channel | Easy Recipes, TV Shows. https://www.foodnetwork.com/.../healthy-mains/food-network-most-saved-healthy-recipes

Frey, M. (2020, October 31). 11 "Bad" Eating Habits You Can Break for Good. Verywell Fit. https://www.verywell-fit.com/how-to-break-bad-eating-habits-for-good-4153595

Healthy Recipes. (n.d.). Allrecipes. Retrieved February 11, 2021, from https://www.allrecipes.com/recipes/84

Healthy Recipes and Ideas for Light Meals. (n.d.). Good Housekeeping. Retrieved February 11, 2021, from https://www.goodhousekeeping.com/food-recipes/healthy

Improving Your Eating Habits. (2019). https://www.cdc.gov/

healthyweight/losing_weight/eating_habits.html

John. (2019, February 22). Bad Eating Habits? Avoiding The Triggers That Hinder A Weight Loss Plan. NJDiet. https://www.njdiet.com/2019/02/22/bad-eating-habits-avoiding-the-triggers-that-hinder...

Livermore, S., & Flager, M. (2020, December 7). Healthy Twists on Your Favorite Comfort Foods. Delish. https://www.delish.com/cooking/recipe-ideas/g3733/healthy-dinner-recipes

MacPherson, R. (2021, January 20). A psychologist offers ways to change bad diet habits. Insider. https://www.insider.com/how-to-change-diet-habits

Mandal, A. (2014). Study of prevalence of type 2 diabetes mellitus and hypertension in overweight and obese people. Journal of Family Medicine and Primary Care, 3(1), 25. https://doi.org/10.4103/2249-4863.130265

McDonald, T. (2021, January 31). How Can I Change My Bad Eating Habits And Lose Weight? Fit.Digital. https://fit.digital/how-can-i-change-my-bad-eating-habits-and-lose-weight

Myshapa. (2018, January 26). 5 Ways to Break Bad Eating Habits For Weight Loss. Shapa Blog. https://blog.myshapa.com/break-bad-eating-habits-weight-loss

NHS Choices. (2019). What are the health benefits of losing weight? NHS. https://www.nhs.uk/common-health-questions/lifestyle/what-are-the-health-benefits-of-losing-weight/

Pathare, S. (2019, August 21). Yoga for Weight Loss: 9 Asanas to Help You Lose Weight. HealthifyMe Blog. https://www.healthifyme.com/blog/yoga-weight-loss-9-asanas/

Saligumba, J. M. (2020, October 11). Gastric Band Hypnosis | Hypnosis | Psychotherapy. Scribd. https://www.scribd.com/document/479570180/Gastric-Band-Hypnosis

Zelman, K. M., MPH, RD, & LD. (n.d.). 6 Steps to Changing Bad Eating Habits. WebMD. https://www.webmd.com/diet/obesity/features/6-steps-to-changing-bad-eating-habits

www.ingramcontent.com/pod-product-compliance
Lightning Source LLC
Chambersburg PA
CBHW071216240726
48654CB00009B/807